NUTRITION AND HEALTH

Edited by

Tanya Carr
BSc SRDR.Nutr
and
Koen Descheemaeker
PhD MBA

Scientific committee

Prof. P. Aggett
Ms M. Brady
Dr. W. Doyle (Observer)
Prof. A. Haines
Prof. M. Hill
Dr. A. Leeds
Dr. B. Margetts
Prof. I. Rowland
Dr. C. Summerbell
Dr. C. Waine

Blackwell
Science

© 2002 by
Blackwell Science Ltd
Editorial Offices:
Osney Mead, Oxford OX2 0EL
25 John Street, London WC1N 2BS
23 Ainslie Place, Edinburgh EH3 6AJ
350 Main Street, Malden
 MA 02148 5018, USA
54 University Street, Carlton
 Victoria 3053, Australia
10, rue Casimir Delavigne
 75006 Paris, France

Other Editorial Offices:

Blackwell Wissenschafts-Verlag GmbH
Kurfürstendamm 57
10707 Berlin, Germany

Blackwell Science KK
MG Kodenmacho Building
7-10 Kodenmacho Nihombashi
Chuo-ku, Tokyo 104, Japan

Iowa State University Press
A Blackwell Science Company
2121 S. State Avenue
Ames, Iowa 50014-8300, USA

First published 2002

Set in 10.5/12.5 pt Garamond Book
by DP Photosetting, Aylesbury, Bucks
Printed and bound in Great Britain by
MPG Books Ltd, Bodmin, Cornwall

DISTRIBUTORS

Marston Book Services Ltd
PO Box 269
Abingdon
Oxon OX14 4YN
(*Orders:* Tel: 01235 465500
 Fax: 01235 465555)

USA and Canada
Iowa State University Press
A Blackwell Science Company
2121 S. State Avenue
Ames, Iowa 50014-8300
(*Orders:* Tel: 800-862-6657
 Fax: 515-292-3348
 Web: www.isupress.com
 email: orders@isupress.com)

Australia
Blackwell Science Pty Ltd
54 University Street
Carlton, Victoria 3053
(*Orders:* Tel: 03 9347 0300
 Fax: 03 9347 5001)

A catalogue record for this title is available
from the British Library

ISBN 0-632-05844-7

Library of Congress
Cataloging-in-Publication Data
is available

For further information on
Blackwell Science, visit our website:
www.blackwell-science.com

For information about future Nutrition and
Health conferences, please contact:

Nutrition and Health Conference
PO Box 24052
London NW4 3ZG
Tel/Fax: 020 8455 2126
Website: www.nutritionandhealth.co.uk
Email: admin@nutritionandhealth.co.uk

CONTENTS

Contents

PREFACE

Every day, new scientific evidence demonstrates that nutrition has an important impact on the health of the individual. Epidemiological studies suggest that specific nutrition habits of various populations can significantly decrease the risk of several chronic diseases.

Scientists have identified a number of components within food, which have important biological activities with potential health benefits. Research is still ongoing but it is becoming apparent that the components within foods and possibly between foods may interact in synergy. This continues to reinforce the message that the consumption of food as a whole is the most ideal way to obtain healthy nutrition.

The researchers are not alone in being convinced about the positive influence of food on health. Amongst health professionals the new knowledge about the relevance of nutrition has spread quickly and is increasingly applied to clinical practice.

In order to highlight the most recent developments in the field of nutrition relevant to dietary advice, we have taken the initiative to organise the Nutrition and Health Conference. This yearly event offers a platform where health professionals can couple theory with practice. It is viewed as a multidisciplinary setting where all health professionals can interact and share ideas. The conference also enables food companies to play an important role in the nutrition and health debate. The enormous interest shown in this conference demonstrates that this domain is in full development and that health professionals are becoming increasingly acquainted with nutrition.

This book contains the lectures which were given at the first Nutrition and Health Conference held in London at the end of 2000. The authors, who are all experts in their fields, give a concise and comprehensive overview on topics related to nutrition and health.

This book is not only designed as a reference for those present at the conference; it is also intended as an informative resource for all who are interested in this discipline and wish to keep pace with the latest developments.

Our sincere thanks go to all the authors.

Tanya Carr
Koen Descheemaeker

CONTRIBUTORS

Paola Albertazzi

She is Clinical Lecturer at the University of Hull, where she works at the Centre for Metabolic Bone Disease. She studied medicine at the University of Bologna in Italy where she graduated with Honours. She has been a Member of the Royal College of Obstetrics and Gynaecology since 1993. Her research is focusing on the effect of drugs and nutrients in several issues of post-menopausal women's health such as bone, indices of cardiovascular disease, and the central nervous system.

Correspondence: Dr. Paola Albertazzi, Clinical Lecturer, Centre for Metabolic Bone Disease, H.S. Brocklehurst Building, Hull Royal Infirmary, 220-236 Anlaby Road, Hull, HU3 2RW, UK.

Email: P.Albertazzi@medschool.hull.ac.uk

Margaret Ashwell

She has viewed the relationship between food, nutrition science and public health from all sides. From her role as Senior Research Scientist with the Medical Research Council, through her role as Principal of the Good Housekeeping Institute and more recently as Science Director of the British Nutrition Foundation and as member of the Government's Food Advisory Committee, she has considered the issues as they affect scientists, consumers, the media, the Government and the food industry. She now runs an independent consultancy, specialising in research co-ordination and dissemination. She is able to use her breadth of experience and novel ideas to work with all sectors and enjoys the variety of challenges that arise.

Correspondence: Dr. Margaret Ashwell OBE, Ashwell Associates, Ashwell Street, Ashwell, Hertfordshire, SG7 5PZ, UK.

Email: ashwell@compuserve.com

Eric Brunner

He is a senior lecturer in the Department of Epidemiology and Public Health at University College London, where he teaches epidemiology. He studied biochemistry and epidemiology, and completed his PhD on social inequalities in coronary disease in 1994. He is a principal investigator on the Whitehall II study and leads the biological and nutritional components. He is active in the evidence-based approach to nutrition and an editor of the Cochrane Heart Group.

Correspondence: Dr Eric Brunner, Department Epidemiology & Public Health, University College London, 1-19 Torrington Place, London WC1E 6BT, UK.

Email: E.Brunner@ucl.ac.uk

Judy Buttriss

She is the British Nutrition Foundation's Science Director, a post she has held for 3 years. She has qualifications in human nutrition and in dietetics and is a Registered Public Health Nutritionist. Her PhD and postdoctoral research work concerned antioxidant vitamins (vitamins C and E), and the mineral selenium. She is Honorary Secretary of the Nutrition Society, visiting Senior Lecturer at Southampton University and a member of a number of committees, including MAFF's National Food Survey Committee and the Expert Group of the Joint Health Claims Initiative.

Correspondence: Dr Judy Buttriss, British Nutrition Foundation, 52-54 High Holborn, London, WC1V 6RQ, UK.

E-mail: j.buttriss@nutrition.org.uk

Anne Dornhurst

She is a consultant diabetologist at the Hammersmith Hospital and Charing Cross Hospital in London. Having graduated from Oxford Medical School she completed her postgraduate and research training in the Johns Hopkins Hospital in the USA. Dr Dornhorst's research interest includes the metabolic changes that occur in pregnancy and the way maternal changes in metabolism influence the growth and development of children and their future susceptibility to obesity and diabetes. Dr Dornhorst has written a number of papers on risk factors that contribute to the development of diabetes following a gestational diabetic pregnancy. Dr Dornhorst is a firm believer that the growing epidemic of diabetes needs to be controlled by public health initiatives that include the adoption of improved diet and exercise programmes.

Correspondence: Dr Anne Dornhorst, Department of Metabolic Medicine Division of Investigative Science, 6th Floor Commonwealth Building, Imperial College School of Medicine, Imperial College at Hammersmith Campus, Du Cane Road, London W12 0NN, UK.

Email: a.dornhurst@ic.ac.uk

Carolyn Edwards

She is a clinical psychologist working at the Health Behaviour Unit at University College London. She is currently involved in the development and evaluation of a cognitive-behavioural treatment programme for weight management.

Correspondence: Dr. Carolyn Edwards, Department of Epidemiology and Public Health, University College London, WC1E 6BT, UK.

Email: c.edwards@public-health.ucl.ac.uk

Stewart Forsyth

He studied at Glasgow University and was awarded The Van den Berghs and Jurgens 1983 Nutrition Award Prize-Winning Paper for his study, 'The Importance of Nutrition in Acute Clinical Care – The Preterm Infant'. In 1992 he was then awarded The Alexander Bryce Nutrition Prize from the

University of Glasgow for his paper, 'Is early solid feeding harmful to the infant?' He is currently Clinical Group Director for the Woman and Child Health Group at Tayside University Hospitals Trust. He is also a Consultant Paediatrician and an Honorary Senior Lecturer for the Department of Health at the University of Dundee. Dr. Forsyth's principal research theme has been the investigation of the relationship of infant nutrition and metabolism to later childhood health and development. However, his most recent research development has focused on investigating the effects of long chain polyunsaturated fatty acid supplementation on infant and cognitive behaviour. He has contributed to over seventy publications and has been the successful recipient or co-recipient of over twenty research grants in excess of £1.5 million.

Correspondence: Dr Stewart Forsyth, Neonatal Intensive Care Unit, Ninewells Hospital, Dundee, Scotland, DD1 9SY, UK.

Email: stewartf@tuht.scot.nhs.uk

Kenneth R. Fox

He is Professor and Head of Department of Exercise and Health Sciences, University of Bristol. His qualifications include a BSc (London), Cert Ed (Loughborough) MSc (Kansas State) and PhD (Arizona State). He serves on the Executive Committee of the Association for the Study of Obesity, and has contributed to the British Nutrition Foundation and National Audit Office Task Forces on Obesity. His research and writing focus on the role of exercise in weight management and mental health.

Correspondence: Professor Ken Fox, Department of Exercise and Health Sciences, Priory House, 8 Woodland Road, Bristol University, Bristol, BS8 1TN, UK.

Email: K.R.Fox@bristol.ac.uk

Gary Frost

He is head of Nutrition and Dietetics at the Hammersmith Hospitals NHS Trust and Honorary Senior Lecturer at Imperial College of Medicine. He studied dietetics at Leeds Metropolitan University until 1982 and completed his PhD at London University in 1996. His research is focusing on the effects of carbohydrate in diabetes and heart disease.

Correspondence: Dr Gary Frost, Department of Nutrition and Dietetic, Hammersmith Hospital, Du Cane Road, London, W12 0HS.

Email: gfrost@hhnt.org

Glenn R. Gibson

He is currently Professor of Food Microbiology and Head of the Food Microbial Sciences Unit at the University of Reading. This is a research unit within the University that is researching gut microbiology and food safety. Prior to that he was head of microbiology at the Institute of Food Research in Reading. He also spent 8 years at the Medical Research Council Dunn Clinical Nutrition Centre in Cambridge. He has published widely on the area of human gut bacteriology. Current research interests include the application of prebiotics for improved health, disease outcomes of gut microbiology and the application of molecular techniques to colonic bacteriology.

Correspondence: Professor GR Gibson, School of Food Biosciences, The University of Reading, Whiteknights, Reading, RG6 6BZ, UK.

Email: g.r.gibson@reading.ac.uk

Michael Hill

He is Professor of Microbial Ecology and Health at South Bank University. His BSc, PhD and DSc were in chemistry from London University. He is also a Fellow of the Royal College of Pathologists and of the Royal Society of Chemistry. He is Chairman of the European Cancer Prevention Organization (ECP), and his main research interests are in diet and human cancer prevention. He is Chairman of the Royal Society of Medicine's Forum on Food and Health.

Correspondence: Professor Michael Hill, Nutrition Research Centre, South Bank University, 103 Borough Road, London, SE1 0AA, UK.

Email: hillmj@sbu.ac.uk

Alan A. Jackson

Alan Jackson is Professor of Human Nutrition in the School of Medicine, University of Southampton. Having trained in paediatrics, he worked on improved methods for the treatment of children with severe malnutrition, the mechanisms through which people adapt to inadequate food and its impact upon development. Current work explores the extent to which modest differences in maternal diet and metabolic competence influence fetal development, predisposing to chronic disease in adulthood. He is involved in the education of clinicians in nutrition, based upon the minimum understanding required to make a doctor safe to practice.

Correspondence: Professor Alan A. Jackson, Institute of Human Nutrition, University of Southampton, Southampton General Hospital (Mailpoint 113), Tremona Road, Southampton, SO16 6YD, UK.

Email: aaj@soton.ac.uk

Jaak Ph. Janssens

He is Professor at the Limburg University Centre of Diepenbeek, and oncologist at the Limburg Oncological Centre, Belgium, and active in the field of oncology, breast cancer and nutrition. He studied medicine and made his PhD in biochemistry in 1985 at the Catholic University of Leuven, Belgium. His research is focusing on environmental and lifestyle factors in breast cancer development. He is a member of several advisory committees related to nutrition and chronic diseases, including the European Cancer Prevention Organization.

Correspondence: Professor J. Ph. Janssens, Biomed Institute, University Campus Building C, Limburg University Centre, 3590 Diepenbeek, Belgium.

Email: janssens.ecp@skynet.be

Susan A. Jebb

She is Head of Nutrition and Health Research at MRC Human Nutrition Research in Cambridge. Her research focuses on the role of dietary factors in the prevention and treatment of obesity and its metabolic comorbidities. She is also Deputy Chair of the UK Association for the Study of Obesity.

Correspondence: Dr Susan Jebb, MRC Human Nutrition Research, Elsie Widdowson Laboratory, Fulbourn Road, Cambridge, CB1 9NL, UK.

Email: Susan.Jebb@mrc-hnr.cam.ac.uk

Ian T. Johnson

He is currently Head of the Diet and the Gastrointestinal Tract Group at the Institute of Food Research, Norwich, and he holds an Honorary Chair in the School of Health at UEA. Having graduated from the University of London with a degree in Zoology and Comparative Physiology he undertook a PhD concerned with the physiology of intestinal folate transport. He then carried out post-doctoral research at the universities of London and York, and joined the Institute of Food Research in Norwich in 1979. The work of his research group continues to be focused on the alimentary tract, the main areas of interest being the relationship between diet and gastrointestinal cancer, and the intestinal absorption of nutrients and phytochemicals.

Correspondence: Professor IT Johnson, Institute of Food Research, Norwich Research Park, Colney, Norwich, NR4 7UA, UK.

Email: ian.johnson@bbsrc.ac.uk

Tim J. Key

He is a senior scientist and reader in epidemiology at the Imperial Cancer Research Fund Cancer Epidemiology Unit, University of Oxford. He studied veterinary medicine, nutrition and epidemiology. His main interests are the roles of diet and sex hormones in the aetiology of cancer, particularly cancers of the breast and prostate. He currently works mostly on the European Prospective Investigation into Cancer and Nutrition (EPIC), as the principal investigator of the Oxford cohort of 60 000 subjects and the chairman of the EPIC prostate cancer group. He is also a member of the UK government's Scientific Advisory Committee on Nutrition.

Correspondence: Dr Tim Key, ICRF Cancer Epidemiology Unit, Gibson Building, Radcliffe Infirmary, Oxford, OX2 6HE, UK.

Email: key@icrf.icnet.uk

Suzi Leather

She is Deputy Chair of the Food Standards Agency, which was established on 1 April 2000. She was Chair of Exeter & District Community Health Trust from December 1997 to April 2001 and has worked in consumer representation since 1978. She is a freelance researcher and writer on consumer aspects of public policy, specialising in health, food and agricultural issues.

Ms Leather has worked at regional, national and European level and is a leading national authority on nutrition and poverty. She was the first Chair of the North & East Devon Health Forum – an inter-agency body with a remit to improve health and tackle health inequalities. Ms Leather also chairs the St Sidwell's project, a healthy living centre focusing on better physical, mental and spiritual health.

Correspondence: Ms Suzi Leather, Food Standards Agency, Room 615C, Aviation House, Holborn, London, WC2B 6NH, UK.

Email: suzi.leather@foodstandards.gsi.gov.uk

Anne M. Molloy

She is a Senior Experimental Officer at Trinity College Dublin where her research is focused on biochemical, nutritional and genetic interactions of folate and vitamin B_{12}. She studied biochemistry at University College Dublin and completed her PhD in Biochemistry in 1980 at Trinity College Dublin.

Correspondence: Dr Anne Molloy, Department of Biochemistry, Trinity College Dublin, Dublin 2, Ireland.

Email: amolloy@tcd.ie

Susan A. New

Dr Susan New is a Registered Public Health Nutritionist and has been a Lecturer in Nutrition within the School of Biomedical & Life Sciences at the University of Surrey since 1996, having previously worked and studied at the University of Aberdeen and the Rowett Research Institute. Her research focuses on the area of nutrition and bone health, for which she has won a number of awards. These include the 1991 UK Nutritional Consultative Panel PhD Scholarship, three Young Investigators Prizes at the 1st World Congress of Osteoporosis (Holland, May 1996), the 7th UK Osteoporosis Conference (Bath, April 2000) and the 1st Joint Meeting of the International Bone & Mineral Society & European Calcified Tissue Society (Madrid June 2001) as well as the 2001 Nutrition Society Medal. She is a Member of the Scientific Advisory Council of the National Osteoporosis Society and the Scientific Advisory Committee of the British Nutrition Foundation. Susan is also the Honorary Communications Officer of the UK Nutrition Society and an Honorary Research Fellow of the Rowett Research Institute.

Correspondence: Dr Susan A. New, Centre for Nutrition & Food Safety, School of Biomedical & Life Sciences, University of Surrey, Guildford, Surrey, GU2 7XH, UK.

Email: s.new@surrey.ac.uk

Stephen Rollnick

He is now Senior Lecturer in the Department of General Practice, University of Wales, College of Medicine. He worked as clinical psychologist in the British National Health Service for 16 years. His background is in the addiction field, where he developed, with William R. Miller, a counselling method called motivational interviewing for using empathic listening in difficult interviews about change.

His current interest is in the more widespread consultation about behaviour change in general health care settings (e.g. diabetes management; cardiac rehabilitation; health promotion; medication adherence; renal disease management, and so on). He has trained practitioners in many countries and continents and has published widely on health care interventions. He has conducted collaborative research with a number of organisations, including the World Health Organization and the National Drug & Alcohol Research Centre in Sydney, Australia. His most recent book is *Health Behavior Change: A Guide for Practitioners* (co-authors Pip Mason & Chris Butler; Churchill Livingstone, 1999).

Correspondence: Dr Stephen Rollnick, Senior Lecturer Department of General Practice University of Wales, College of Medicine, Llanedeyrn Health Centre, Llanedeyrn, Cardiff, CF3 7PN, UK.

Email: rollnick@cf.ac.uk

Imogen Sharp

She is Head of the Coronary Heart Disease and Stroke Prevention Branch at the Department of Health, responsible for policy on nutrition, physical activity and obesity. She was formerly Director of the National Heart Forum, where she published a number of documents including *Social Inequalities in Coronary Heart Disease: Opportunities for Action* (1998) and *At Least Five a Day: Strategies to Increase Fruit and Vegetable Consumption* (1997). She has a BSc (Hons) in Human sciences and an MSc in Health Planning and Financing, and previously taught behavioural sciences at the University of Hong Kong Medical School.

Correspondence: Ms Imogen Sharp, Department of Health, Wellington House, 133–155 Waterloo Road, London SE1 8UG, UK.

Email: DHMail@doh.gsi.gov.uk

Susan Southon

She is Professor and Head of Micronutrients at the Institute of Food Research (IFR), UK. She gained first class honours in Biological Sciences at Lancaster University, followed by a PhD in nutrient metabolism. After several years' research in mineral nutrition, she diversified into vitamins and now leads a wide range of projects on absorption, metabolism and bioactivity of folate vitamers and carotenoids. She has been successful in the co-ordination of EU research projects encompassing issues from farm to fork, and fork to function in humans.

Correspondence: Professor Susan Southon, Institute of Food Research, Norwich Research Park, Colney, Norwich, NR4 7UA, UK.

Email: sue.southon@bbsrc.ac.uk

Gilbert R. Thompson

He is Emeritus Professor in Clinical Lipidology, Imperial College School of Medicine and led the Medical Research Council Lipoprotein Team at Hammersmith Hospital, where he was Honorary Consultant Physician in charge of the Lipid Clinic, until his retirement. His research is mainly on lipoprotein metabolism and atherosclerosis, and he is a past-chairman of both the British Hyperlipidaemia Association and the British Athero-sclerosis Society.

Correspondence: Professor Gilbert Thompson, Metabolic Medicine, ICSM, Hammersmith Hospital, Du Cane Rd, London, W12 0NN, UK.

Email: g.thompson@ic.ac.uk

Pieter van't Veer

Dr Pieter van't Veer, PhD, is associate professor in the Nutritional Epi-demiology of Cancer. He studied Human Nutrition at Wageningen University, The Netherlands, and Epidemiology at Harvard University, Boston. His research focused on cancer of the breast, colon and liver, and is currently extended to prostate cancer. The use of biomarkers to improve the assessment of the biologically relevant exposure into observational studies on diet and cancer has been central to his work.

Correspondence: Dr P. van't Veer, Division of Human Nutrition and Epi-demiology, Wageningen University, PO Box 8129, 6700 EV Wageningen, The Netherlands.

Email: pieter.vantveer@staff.nutepi.wau.nl

Geoff Watts

Geoff Watts read zoology at King's College, London. He moved into medical research and completed a PhD before leaving the academic world for science and medical journalism. For many years he presented the BBC Radio 4 programme *Medicine Now*. He now presents a weekly science programme *Leading Edge*, and divides his time between broadcasting, writing and speaking. He is member of the Government's Human Genetics Commission.

Correspondence: Dr Geoff Watts, 28 New End Square, London, NW3 1LS, UK.

Email: geoff@scileg.freeserve.co.uk

Gary Williamson

He is Professor and head of the Phytochemicals Group, Institute of Food Research (IFR), UK. He studied biochemistry and completed his PhD in Sheffield in 1983. His research interests are dietary phytochemicals – health implications (beneficial and toxic) and exploitation, including bioavailability of non-nutrient antioxidants especially polyphenols and glucosinolates. His current research focuses on the fate, activity and metabolism of phytochemicals at all stages of consumption and how this is related to enzyme specificity.

Correspondence: Professor Gary Williamson, Head of Phytochemicals Team, Nutrition Health and Consumer Sciences Division, Institute of Food Research, Norwich Research Park, Colney, Norwich, NR4 7UA, UK.

Email: gary.williamson@bbsrc.ac.uk

INTRODUCTION

PREVENTION, A GOVERNMENT PRIORITY

IMOGEN SHARP

For this government, preventing and reducing health inequalities is of vital importance. The NHS Plan, the NHS Cancer Plan and the National Service Framework for Coronary Heart Disease recognise cancer and coronary heart disease as major priorities – focusing not only on the clinical but also the preventive aspects of the disease.

By tackling the major risk factors for these chronic diseases, such as smoking and nutrition, early deaths can be reduced. Recognising the links between diet and later disease, the NHS Plan highlights diet and nutrition as a key area for action.

Evidence

Evidence shows that eating at least five portions of fruit and vegetables a day could lead to estimated reductions of up to 20% in overall deaths from chronic diseases such as heart disease, stroke and cancer. Experts suggest that it is the second most effective strategy to reduce the risk of cancer, after reducing smoking.

Yet, on average, adults are eating only 250 g, around three portions a day, while children are eating only two portions a day. These average figures mask wide variation between individuals:

- unskilled groups eat about 50% less than professional groups
- children in the lowest income groups are about 50% less likely to eat fruit and vegetables than those in the highest income groups

- one in five children (20%) eat no fruit at all in a week
- nearly 70% of 2–12 year olds consume biscuits, sweets or chocolate at least once a day.

Strong social gradients are also found in intakes of vitamin C and folate, with lower intakes among lower income groups.

The NHS plan (2000)

People make their own choices about what to eat. It is the role of government to ensure they have information and proper access to a healthy diet, wherever they live. So by 2004, it is planned to have in place:

- the National School Fruit Scheme
- Welfare Foods Programme reform to ensure children in poverty have access to a healthy diet
- increased support for breastfeeding
- a five-a-day programme to increase fruit and vegetable consumption; a communications programme will begin in 2001
- improved access to fruit and vegetables through local initiatives working with industry; five community pilot sites were launched in October 2000
- reduce salt, sugar and fat in diet, working with industry and the Food Standards Agency
- local action to tackle obesity and physical inactivity, informed by advice from the Health Development Agency. Most adults in England are now overweight, and one in five is obese
- a hospital nutrition policy to improve the outcome of care for patients.

Five-a-day programme

A five-a-day programme to increase fruit and vegetable consumption and help make a healthy diet a real choice for everyone is being developed. This includes:

- National School Fruit Scheme
- Five-a-day Community Projects
- a communications programme
- working with industry to improve provision and access
- evaluation and monitoring.

We cannot develop the programme alone, therefore we are liaising with a number of key stakeholders to increase provision of and access to fruit and vegetables:

- other government departments and agencies – Food Standards Agency, Ministry of Agriculture, Fisheries and Food, Department of Employment and Education, and the Health Development Agency
- the food industry – producers, retailer, caterers
- consumer, health and education organisations.

National School Fruit Scheme

The National School Fruit Scheme is an ambitious undertaking. The first government-funded scheme of its kind in the world, it will eventually entail distributing around 400 million pieces of fruit to some 16 000 infant schools across England each year. This is equivalent to 40% of the British apple market.

It is a huge logistical challenge and so we are examining the practicalities of the scheme through pilots before rolling it out nationally. There are three aspects to consider:

- farm to school gate – getting the fruit delivered to schools
- school gate to child's hand – distributing fruit in the school
- child's hand to mouth – encouraging children to eat the fruit.

Already the pilot schemes are providing a free piece of fruit to around 80 000 children in over 500 schools across England every day.

Five-a-day Community Projects

The Five-a-day Community Projects, as highlighted in the Cancer Plan (2000), started in September 2000. They have been set up to develop a coordinated approach to increase fruit and vegetable consumption across a whole community. The projects are testing the feasibility and practicalities of evidence-based community approaches in low-income areas.

A total of one million people are being targeted in five areas across England, in Airedale and Craven, County Durham, Hastings, Sandwell and Somerset. Some of the interventions include working with food retailers and farmers' markets and setting up food cooperatives and a delivery service for those most in need. The lessons learned from these pilot projects will be used to inform the five-a-day programme. The national roll-out will begin in 2002.

Communications programme

A communications programme is being developed to increase awareness of fruit and vegetable consumption. Working with industry, the Food Standards Authority (FSA) and other partners, this will involve the creation of an identity. A primary consideration in the development of this programme will be effective approaches and methods for reaching and influencing low-income groups.

Working with industry

We will be working with industry including producers, caterers and retailers to increase provision of and access to fruit and vegetables.

Evaluation and monitoring

Evaluation and monitoring is a major component of the programme. We will be focusing on the implementation and impact of the five-a-day programme.

National Service Framework for coronary heart disease (CHD)

The National Service Framework for coronary heart disease also sets milestones to improve diet and nutrition:

- reduce heart disease in the population
- prevent CHD in high risk patients in primary care
- reduce risk of subsequent cardiac problems of those already suffering from CHD, and promote their return to a full and normal life.

By April 2001, all NHS bodies will have agreed and be contributing to the delivery of local programmes of effective policies on reducing smoking, promoting healthy eating, increasing physical activity and reducing overweight and obesity. By April 2002, there will be quantitative data about the implementation of these policies.

1

DIET FOR THE PREVENTION OF HEART DISEASE: HOW FAR ARE WE?

ERIC BRUNNER

On the right track

There is a downward trend in coronary heart disease (CHD) mortality in affluent societies including the UK and other countries of Western Europe. CHD mortality peaked in the early 1970s. Since then, the rate of premature coronary mortality has declined by 49% (1972-97 age 35-74: men 554 - 276; women 184 - 100 per 100 000 (WHO data)). Despite the fall of some 2% per year in the CHD death rate over the past quarter century there were over 50 000 premature CHD deaths in the UK in 1998, and the disease remains responsible for more deaths than any other single cause. There has been a similar downward trend in stroke death rates.

Taking cardiovascular disease as a whole (heart and circulatory system including stroke), the death rate for adults under 75 fell from about 270 to 140 per 100 000 between 1970 and 1997. If the present trend continues, the rate will have fallen below the target (80/100 000) for 2010 set in *Our Healthier Nation*.

The CHD death rate among women is about half that among men. This gender difference is poorly understood. It is not limited to the UK, and does not appear to be culturally specific. Paradoxically, women report more chest pain (angina pectoris) than men but are less likely to have electrocardiographic (ECG) abnormalities detected (Nicholson *et al.*, 1999). Nevertheless, women who have angina have an increased risk of heart attack.

Lower socio-economic position is a major determinant of the risk of CHD. There is a stepwise increase in CHD mortality rate with each step down the social strata. A stepwise gradient, rather than poverty threshold effect, is seen whether the social classification used is income, occupation or education. In England and Wales inequalities in CHD mortality widened between 1970 and 1990. Over that period the overall CHD mortality rate declined (see above). If these two observations are put together an important policy problem emerges. Absolute risk of CHD death is declining faster in higher socio-economic groups than in the lower, accounting for the reduction in risk seen in the aggregated national data. But the relative difference in risk across social strata is increasing and thus inequality grows.

Ethnicity is linked with risk for CHD. In the UK, analyses of death certificates according to country of birth show ethnic minorities have greatly differing risks of CHD (Wild & McKeigue, 1997). Afro-Caribbeans are around 40% less likely, and South Asians about 50% more likely to die of heart disease than the 'native' born population. Recent research shows that both ethnic groups have a tendency towards glucose intolerance and insulin resistance, and that type 2 diabetes is relatively common (Whitty *et al.*, 1999). Other cardiovascular risk factors show differences. South Asians tend to have an adverse lipid profile (high serum triglycerides and low HDL-cholesterol), while Afro-Caribbeans do not and are predisposed to high blood pressure and stroke, rather than to CHD. The link between ethnicity and cardiovascular risk is not a fixed one. For example the Japanese in Japan have a very low risk of heart attack, but migrants to the USA quickly develop a CHD risk level similar to the host population. There is debate among researchers about the extent to which the differences in disease risk are cultural, socio-economic or biological in origin. Dietary pattern plays an important role, for example as a determinant of obesity, in Afro-Caribbeans and South Asians.

Current population dietary targets for England include reductions in average total and saturated fat intake, and an increase in fruit and vegetable intake:

- To reduce the average percentage of food energy derived from fat to no more than 35% by the year 2005
- To reduce the average percentage of food energy derived from saturated fat to no more than 11% by the year 2005
- To increase the consumption of fruit and vegetables by 50%.

The targets for fat are from *Health of the Nation* (1996) and are being reviewed. The target for fruit and vegetables (Committee on Medical Aspects of Food Policy, 1994) is similar to that recommended by the same policy committee for the prevention of cancer, specifically colorectal and gastric cancers, and tentatively, breast cancer. In the case of cancer, COMA recommended simply that 'fruit and vegetable consumption in the UK should increase' (Committee on Medical Aspects of Food Policy, 1998).

Partial progress towards these public health targets has been made (MAFF, 1999). Over the past decade (1988–1998) the proportion of food energy derived from fat declined by 8% (from 42% to 39%) while that derived from saturated fatty acids declined by 12% (from 17% to 15%). In 1992, shortly before the fruit and vegetable target was set, average adult consumption (excluding potatoes and potato products) was just under 300 g per person per day, while in 1998 it was just above, at some 310 g, corresponding to an average increase in consumption of 7%, or about 3 g per person per year.

Table 1.1 shows estimates of the weekly consumption of fresh fruit and vegetables in 1998, excluding potatoes, according to household income group and employment status. It is evident that the higher levels of fruit and vegetable consumption are linked with higher socio-economic position, and that pensioners are perhaps more diet conscious than adults in younger households.

Table 1.1   Fresh fruit and vegetable consumption according to weekly income of head of household, and among pensioners, 1998 (gram/person/week).

	<£160	£160–£329	£330–£639	£640+	No earner, <£160	OAP
Fresh fruit	505	606	704	964	588	835
Fresh vegetables*	536	648	726	899	621	894

* excluding potatoes
OAP = Old age pensioner households
Source: National Food Survey 1998.

What we have learnt

Geoffrey Rose, an articulate advocate of prevention, wrote that 'politicians influence health more than the doctors' (Rose, 1992). He recognised that fiscal and regulatory measures are an essential part of an effective policy on food and health. For example, the Food Standards Agency is playing a pivotal role in tackling microbiological and other problems, and restoring confidence in the food supply, by legislative means.

Rose recognised that if there was an approximate linear relationship between the exposure level (e.g. saturated fat intake) and the associated risk of disease, then the optimal preventive strategy will be to seek to shift the population distribution of risk downwards ('to the left') because the greater part of the disease burden occurs among those who are around the centre of the distribution of intake, and not among those with the highest intakes. The same principle applies to protective foods such as fruit and vegetables, except that in such cases the policy aim is to shift the population distribution of risk upwards ('to the right').

In the classic case of serum cholesterol and coronary disease, risk increases as the serum cholesterol level goes up. However, serum cholesterol has a normal, bell-shaped, distribution and a relatively small proportion of the UK population has a very high serum cholesterol level. Therefore, most cases of the disease occur in those with only moderately raised blood cholesterol, because there are far more individuals in the centre of the distribution than at the extreme. The appropriate public health response to such problems of widespread risk is to reduce risk in the population as a whole, rather than to target only the high-risk group and thus miss most of those who will develop disease. The health services can then focus efforts on helping the highest risk individuals.

The strategy of prevention described above is appropriate to the prevention of hypertension, stroke and CHD by means of reduction in salt intake. Most salt is consumed in non-discretionary forms, and the Department of Health is asking food manufacturers to develop product formulations with a smaller salt content in order to shift the sodium intake distribution downwards. This policy is based on comparisons of a variety of population studies such as Intersalt and trials of salt restriction which demonstrate over the medium term (in the absence of long-term trials) that habitual salt intake is an important and modifiable determinant of blood pressure in healthy people (Brunner *et al.*, 1997; Cutler *et al.*, 1997).

Dietary advice provided by health professionals appears to be modestly effective in promoting changes in food intake in the general population. Those who are sick or have raised risk factor levels, as might be expected, are well motivated to make salutogenic changes; however even among healthy people, dietary advice does appear to have positive effects

(Brunner *et al.*, 1997). A systematic review of controlled trials of dietary advice of nine months or longer provides realistic estimates of the likely changes. These include net reductions of some 0.22 mM (3.7%) in serum cholesterol, 45 mmol/24 h (29%) in urinary sodium excretion and 1.2 mmHg (1.4%) in diastolic blood pressure. Assuming the diet-related reductions in serum cholesterol and diastolic BP are sustained, CHD and stroke incidence would fall by an estimated 14% and 8% respectively. These risk reductions are valuable, given the multi-factorial origins of cardiovascular disease.

In addition to individual dietary advice, improving the food supply appears to be a cost effective approach to dietary change (Brunner *et al.*, 2001a, b). A good example is the increase in intake of polyunsaturated fatty acids (PUFA), which took place in England in the 1980s. During that decade the ratio of PUFA to saturated fatty acids (PS ratio) in the average diet almost doubled as a result of the increased availability of inexpensive vegetable and seed oils, and palatable high-PUFA margarines. The change in PS ratio is likely to have contributed to the observed reduction in serum cholesterol in the general population.

Dietary advice in the 1970s placed considerable emphasis on reduction of total fat intake as a key to CHD prevention. According to the National Food Survey this has been achieved in part, to the extent that over the past decade average fat intake has dropped by some 8%. This is likely to have contributed to the reduction in CHD mortality rates. Additionally, several lines of evidence suggest that simultaneous changes in the composition of dietary fat, particularly the reduction in mean saturated fatty acid intake and the increase in unsaturated fatty acid intake, have had comparable benefits for cardiovascular health. Clarke *et al.* (1997) estimate, on the basis of short-term metabolic ward studies, that replacement of 10% of dietary energy from saturates by mono- and polyunsaturated fatty acids reduces serum cholesterol by some 13% (from 6.0 to 5.2 mmol/l). This compares with a reduction in CHD events, estimated from reviews of dietary intervention trials, of 14% (Brunner *et al.*, 1997) to 17% (Truswell, 1994). CHD mortality has halved in the past 25 years.

Unsolved problems

Valuable advances in our understanding of population nutrition have come in the twentieth century. At the beginning of the twenty-first century, problems remaining to be solved include the astonishing increase in prevalence of overweight and obesity, and the question of the optimal diet for today's living conditions. The issue of overweight and obesity is dealt with in Chapter 7. Related to the problem of obesity is the question of the optimal diet for preventing obesity and metabolic complications such as glucose intolerance and an atherogenic blood lipid profile. An important research objective is to examine whether saturated fat is best replaced with carbohydrate or unsaturated fat, or a mixture of both. Observational data from the Whitehall II study (Brunner, 2001b) provide evidence that both PUFA and carbohydrate offer metabolic benefits, with few adverse effects, compared with saturated fats.

Taking nutrition further: evidence-based nutrition

My view for the future of nutrition in the twenty-first century is to develop the subject with a population-based approach, drawing from epidemiological and evidence-based medicine. Key perspectives are summarised here.

(1) *Knowledge not information.* While primary research continues to be the main focus of academic nutrition, there is a relative weakness in extracting knowledge from the existing body of research findings.
(2) *Systematic not narrative reviews.* A paradigm shift is needed in nutrition. Narrative reviews are journalistic, subjective, and even impressionistic. Consideration needs to be given to the possibility that systematic reviews would be more valuable building blocks for future research and the application of existing findings.
(3) *Heterogeneity not dissent.* Debates in nutrition, for example, on the question of carbohydrate versus PUFA or monounsaturated fats as substitute for energy from saturated fatty acids currently tend to be based on argument from a fixed scientific viewpoint, using statements that may begin 'The latest study shows...'. It is possible that more rapid progress may be made by attempting to understand the reasons for the heterogeneity of results within a systematic review, rather than focusing on consensus and dissent.

References

Brunner, E., White, I.R., Thorogood, M., Bristow, A., Curle, D. & Marmot, M.G. (1997) Can dietary interventions change diet and cardiovascular risk factors? A meta-analysis of randomized controlled trials. *Am. J. Public Health*, **87**, 1415–22.
Brunner, E., Cohen, D., & Toon, L. (2001a) Cost effectiveness of cardiovascular disease prevention strategies a perspective on EU food based dietary guidelines. *Public Health Nutr.* (in press).
Brunner, E., Wunsch, H. & Marmot, M.G. (2001b) What is an optimal diet? Rela-

tionship of macronutrient intake to obesity, glucose tolerance, lipoprotein cholesterol levels and the metabolic syndrome in the Whitehall II study. *Int. J. Obes.* Relat. Metab. Disorder. **25** (1), 45-53.

Clarke, R., Frost, C., Collins, R., Appleby, P. & Peto, R. (1997) Dietary lipids and blood cholesterol: quantitative meta-analysis of metabolic ward studies. *BMJ*, **314**, 112-17.

Committee on Medical Aspects of Food Policy (1994) *Nutritional aspects of cardiovascular disease*. The Stationery Office, London.

Committee on Medical Aspects of Food Policy (1998) *Nutritional aspects of the development of cancer*. The Stationery Office, London.

Cutler, J.A., Follmann, D., & Allender, P.S. (1997) Randomised trials of sodium reduction: an overview, *Am. J. Clin. Nutr.*, **65**, 643S-651S.

Dept of Health (1996) *The Health of the Nation: Technical Supplement*. DoH, London.

MAFF (1999) *National Food Survey*. The Stationery Office, London.

Nicholson, A., White, I., MacFarlane, P., Brunner, E. & Marmot, M. (1999) Rose questionnaire angina in younger men and women: gender differences in the relationship to cardiovascular risk factors and other reported symptoms. *J. Clin. Epidemiol.*, **52**, 337-46.

Rose, G. (1992) *The Strategy of Preventive Medicine*. Oxford University Press, Oxford.

Truswell, A.S. (1994) Review of dietary intervention studies: effect on coronary events and on total mortality. *Aust. N.Z. J. Med.*, **24**, 98-106.

Whitty, C.J.M., Brunner, E., Shipley, M.J., Hemingway, H. & Marmot, M.G. (1999) Differences in biological risk factors for cardiovascular disease between three ethnic groups in the Whitehall II study. *Atherosclerosis*, **142**, 279-86.

Wild, S. & McKeigue, P. (1997) Cross sectional analysis of mortality by country of birth in England and Wales, 1970-92. *B.M.J.*, **314**, 705-10.

2

SHOULD WE EAT FOODS OR BITS OF FOODS? – RELEVANCE TO CARDIOVASCULAR DISEASE

SUSAN SOUTHON

What information is readily available to the consumer on this issue?

Living in a city, consuming commercially processed foods, breathing polluted air, or being 'microwaved' from above by satellites, is endangering your cardiovascular system. Solution? Take Formula X! Formula X supplies the body with ample amounts of antioxidants. It is a proven, easy, time-tested, safe and an effective way to prevent, or even reverse, atherosclerosis.

These words are paraphrased from the kind of information readily obtained on the Internet when antioxidants and heart disease are entered into a search engine. We are also told that wrinkles, absentmindedness, cancer and clogged arteries result from oxidative stress; no single food, or supplement, can help with the oxidative stress associated with modern living; and that a broad-spectrum supplement of antioxidants is essential to minimise degenerative disease. In addition to supplements of anti-oxidant nutrients like vitamins C, E and the carotenoids, we are also exhorted to consider the efficacy of other non-nutrient antioxidants in the form of concentrated herbal extracts, grape extracts and pycnogenol (an extract from the bark of the French maritime pine tree) to name but a few.

Such advertisements, often appearing to the surfer as public information pieces, are laden with words such as 'tested', 'effective', 'safe', 'essential', 'proven'. The information accompanying these products is clear and decisive, while the world of 'real' nutritional science is often muddy and indecisive – full of 'possibly', 'might', 'maybe', 'it is hypothesised' and 'it is suggested' – or frankly contradictory views and results. The following two quotes provide an example of this apparent contradiction. The first comes from a paper in the Journal of the American College of Cardiology (Mosca *et al.*, 1997) that relates to a study of antioxidant vitamins and risk factors for cardiovascular disease (CVD):

> 'These results back-up the findings of previous studies and point to a positive role for antioxidant supplementation among those suffering from coronary artery disease.'

The second quote is from an article in *Circulation*, the Journal of the American Heart Association (Krauss *et al.*, 2000), and again relates to antioxidants and chronic disease.

> 'Current evidence is not strong enough to recommend antioxidant vitamin pills.'

These quotes, apart from highlighting apparently contradictory views of scientists on a very similar point, also serve as an example of the fact that, whilst the science of the public health significance of antioxidant nutrition has developed substantially from observations of people eating traditional diets (some of which appear to substantially protect them from cardiovascular disease (CVD)), research and information is dominated by the supplementation story. The issue of the role of wholefoods consumed within traditional diets versus bits of foods consumed as supplements, or as fortified/functional foods, with regard to the health of the individual consumer, needs debate.

Dietary change

Recent surveys in Europe indicate that far more people are concerned about their food and their health than in the past. However, while consumers say they want to eat healthier, the reality is that they want to eat easier, hence the enormous market potential for dietary supplements, nutrient enriched foods and so called 'functional' foods (Food Industry News, 2000), each of which contain perhaps just one, or just a few, of the thousands of components we consume as part of a normal mixed diet. Compounds isolated from foods, or synthetic copies of compounds that can be found in foods, are promoted and used for their putative medicinal, or health promoting properties. The literature that accompanies their sale can be very convincing to those who want to stay healthy. And for those with a diagnosed condition, these compounds can appear a more natural, and safer, alternative to drug therapy and certainly a much easier option than trying to change dietary habits of a lifetime. Eating more good 'bits' added to foods we like means we do not have to learn to change the dietary habits (perhaps) of a lifetime.

The epidemiology

When developing products that contain higher levels of the supposedly healthy bits of our diet, the choice of what beneficial component, or components, to use is often based on epidemiology, which provides data indicating significant associations between dietary habits, or consumption of specific foods, and reduced risk of a range of chronic diseases. Figure 2.1 shows male coronary incidence in Europe per 100 000 of the population (Tunstall-Pedoe *et al.*, 1999). This graph illustrates very obvious differences in CVD rates in different EU countries, from 200 per 100 000 of the population in Spain to 800 per 100 000 of the population (four times the level) in the UK. If the assumption is correct that these differences in CVD incidence are in large part related to lifestyle factors, including diet, then it follows that a high proportion of the CVD incidences in UK males are potentially avoidable.

In the twentieth century, epidemiologists have been very active providing the experimental scientist with clues as to what types of traditional diet

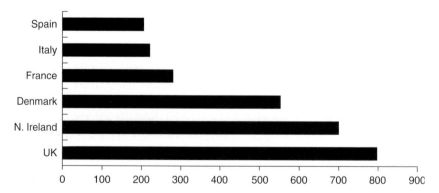

Figure 2.1 Annual coronary-event rate in men, per 100 000 of the population, in 6 European countries; adapted from WHO MONICA Study (Tunstall-Pedoe *et al.*, 1999).

may be involved in decreasing chronic disease risk, particularly CHD and cancer. But we have now entered the brave new world of the twenty-first century. Could nutritional/medical science, food technology and the agro-food industry as a whole, make a contribution to better health into later life using these epidemiological clues as a basis for identifying specific dietary components which might act as 'magic bullets' against specific chronic disease such as CHD?

The exploitation of epidemiological data

Epidemiological data reveals that diets rich in particular foods are associated with reduced risk of a chronic disorder (Gey, 1994). At this stage, however, the association between diet and health is merely an observation. This observation needs then to lead to some reasonable hypothesis, possibly based on earlier experimental evidence. This hypothesis needs to be tested in a wider range of experimental systems, often in vitro and/or animal and cell-line model systems, followed by smaller studies involving human volunteers, perhaps leading to very much larger trials. As part of this process both dose and risk:benefit analysis considerations are vital.

Now the real world of product promotion and profit impinges on the process. Waiting for sound, scientific conclusions and consensus, based upon extensive research, takes time, often a considerable length of time, whilst the need for market edge provides a strong impetus for speedy product development. In developing such products the progression from observation to hypothesis, hypothesis to experimentation in a range of systems, dose response consideration and exploitation of the knowledge gained might be replaced by the leap in the dark strategy. Here the observation is taken directly as the basis on which to develop a product.

A second strategy involves a leap of faith. Here there may be what appears to be sound hypotheses, and experimental data produced using laboratory animals and/or cell cultures. There may still be uncertainty as to the relevance of these data with regard to the human situation, or the dose at which a benefit, or risk, might occur, or if the compounds tested are those which ultimately reach a target site within the human body after digestion, absorption and metabolism.

In both cases, the consumer who buys the product is unwittingly taking part in a potentially very large human study that is poorly controlled and not monitored in any convincing way. But is there reason for concern? Possibly. The carotenoid story serves as an example.

Carotenoid isolates v carotenoid-rich foods

The predominant carotenoids in blood and tissues are:

- β-carotene found in carrots, some orange coloured fruits and green vegetables
- β-cryptoxanthin found in oranges
- lycopene found in tomatoes
- lutein found in yellow/green vegetables.

These compounds have significant antioxidant activity, at least in vitro, and are therefore thought capable of protecting the cells and tissues of our body against the ravages of living in a world full of potentially toxic oxygen (Packer, 1993). Oxidative reactions appear to be intimately associated with atherosclerosis via the oxidation of low-density lipoprotein (LDL) that, when oxidised, is accumulated by macrophage cells in the arterial intima. These lipid-laden macrophages are characteristic of arterial fatty streaks. Antioxidants within LDL, primarily vitamin E and the carotenoids, appear to increase LDL oxidation resistance and, thus, these compounds are hypothesised to prevent or delay the development of atherosclerosis (Halliwell & Gutteridge, 1989).

Carotenoids also have a range of other biological activities. They modulate immune and inflammatory response and have long been known to influence cell-cell communication, which is a vital part of our ability to control the activity of individual cells within a tissue. In vitro and animal studies strongly support some carotenoids as a natural anti-cancer agent, and populations consuming higher amounts of carotenoid-rich foods have lower rates of CVD, cancer and other chronic diseases (van den Berg *et al.*, 2000). There are convincing hypotheses as to why this should be but little is known about what dose provides optimum protection, or how this may vary depending upon individual sensitivity.

Despite this lack of knowledge, human trials were undertaken (Heinonen & Huttonen, 1994; Omenn *et al.*, 1996). Volunteers were given relatively high dose supplements of β-carotene for several years, which raised and maintained a plasma concentration up to tenfold higher than baseline. These studies showed one of two things, either supplementation with β-carotene was not effective with regard to CVD, cancer or all-cause mortality or, in susceptible individuals like smokers and asbestos workers, the mortality rate from lung cancer was significantly increased. On the other hand, plasma β-carotene concentration (reflecting the consumption of carotenoid-rich foods) before supplementation was inversely and significantly associated with lower disease, in this case cancer.

Relatively little 'food', as opposed to 'supplement', experimental research is undertaken. As part of an EU funded study, both isolated carotenoid and carotenoid-rich foods were investigated with respect to their potential benefit with regard to assumed risk factors for atherosclerosis. One risk factor studied was the susceptibility of low-density lipoprotein to oxidation in vitro. In studies of healthy, adult human volunteers, 16 weeks of supplementation with the carotenoids β-carotene, lutein or lycopene had no observable effect on the resistance of human LDL to oxidation. However, after two weeks' supplementation of the diet with additional fruits and vegetables, plasma carotenoids increased significantly, as did LDL oxidation resistance (by approximately 28% in non-smokers and 14% in smokers) (Hininger *et al.*, 1997; Southon, 2000). In addition, as part of this EU study, it was found that oxidised bases in DNA, extracted from the white blood cells of human volunteers, were negatively correlated with serum total carotenoids (Collins *et al.*, 1998); carotenoid supplementation, however, was without further effect (Southon, 2000). Was it the delivery of carotenoids in the correct dose and balance within foods that was responsible for the positive response? Possibly. Was it the effect of carotenoids, plus the many other antioxidant compounds found within the fruits and vegetables that was responsible for the response? Probably.

Vitamin E – prevention or cure?

As with the carotenoids, epidemiology has implicated vitamin E as protective, particularly with respect to CVD (Gey & Puska, 1989). Human intervention studies, involving high dose supplementation, in 'at-risk' individuals, however, have not convincingly demonstrated a role for the vitamin (Riemersma *et al.*, 1989; Heinonen & Huttunen, 1994; Ness & Smith, 1999; Stone, 2000) but perhaps too much is expected. Research has concentrated on the potential for isolated food components to reverse existing disease, whilst the primary role of these food components (in the balance and amounts found in apparently 'protective' diets) is, arguably, most likely to be in the prevention, or slowing, of initiating events.

Brief conclusions and research strategy

Should we eat foods or bits of foods? Epidemiology or pharmacy?

Evidence, albeit largely observational, weighs heavily in favour of the protective effects of specific foods or food groups consumed as part of a traditional diet and a concerted effort should be made to redress the imbalance between whole-food and high dose, single compound research.

Prevention or cure?

Experimental evidence for diet-health relationships is often sought using disease-state models, but appropriate nutrition is far more likely to play a role in prevention rather than cure and the types of experimental models devised need to reflect this.

References

Collins, A., Olmedilla, B., Southon, S., Torbergsen, A., Duthie, S., van den Berg, H., Corridan, B., Hiniger, I. & Thurnham, D. (1998) Carotenoids and oxidative DNA damage, in vivo and ex vivo protective effects in human lymphocytes. *Carcinogenesis*, **19**, 2159-62.

Food Industry News, January 2000, p. 4.

Gey, K.K. (1994) The relationship of antioxidant status and risk of cancer and cardiovascular disease: A critical evaluation of observational data. In: *Free Radicals in the Environment, Medicine and Toxicology* (eds H. Nohl, H. Esterbauer, C. Rice-Evans, pp. 181-219). Richelieu Press, London.

Gey, K.F., & Puska, P. (1989) Plasma vitamins E and A inversely correlated to mortality from ischemic heart disease in cross-cultural epidemiology. *Ann. N.Y. Acad. Sci.*, **570**, 268-82.

Halliwell, B., & Gutteridge, J.M.C. (1989) Free radicals, ageing and disease. In: *Free Radicals in Biology and Medicine*. Clarendon Press, Oxford.

Heinonen, O.P., & Huttunen, J.K. (1994) The effect of vitamin E and beta-carotene on the incidence of lung cancer and other cancers in male smokers. *N. Eng. J. Med.*, **330**, 1029-35.

Hininger, I., Chopra, M., Thurnham, D.I., Laporte, F., Richard, M-J., Favier, A. & Roussel, A-M. (1997) Effect of increased fruit and vegetable intake on the susceptibility of lipoprotein to oxidation. *Eur. J. Clin. Nutr.*, **51**, 601-6.

Krauss, R.M., Eckel, R.H., Howard, B., Appel, L.J., Daniels, S.R., Deckelbaum, R.J. *et al.* (2000) AHA dietary guidelines: revision 2000: A statement for healthcare professionals from the nutrition committee of the American Heart Association, *Circulation*, **102**, 2284-99.

Mosca, L., Rubenfire, M., Mandel, C., Rock , C., Tarshis-Tsai, A., & Pearson T. (1997) Antioxidant nutrient supplementation reduces the susceptibility of low density lipoprotein to oxidation in patients with coronary artery disease. *J. Am. Coll. Cardiol.*, **30**, 392-7.

Ness, A., & Smith, G.D. (1999) Mortality in the CHAOS trial. Cambridge Heart Antioxidant Study, *Lancet*, **20** (353), 1017-18.

Omenn, G.S., Goodman, G.E., Thorquist, M.D., *et al.* (1996) Risk factors for lung cancer and for intervention effects in CARET, the beta-carotene and retinol efficacy trial. *J. Natl. Cancer Inst.*, **88**, 1550-59.

Packer, L. (1993) Antioxidant action of carotenoids in vitro and in vivo and protection against oxidation of human low-density lipoprotein. In: *Carotenoids in Human Health* (eds L.M. Canfield, N.I. Krinsky, J.A. Olsen). New York Academy of Sciences, New York.

Riemersma, R.A., Wood, D.A., Macintyre, C.C., Elton, R., Gey, K.F. & Oliver, M.F. (1989) Low plasma vitamins E and C. Increased risk of angina in Scottish men, *Ann. N.Y. Acad. Sci.*, **570**, 291-5.

Stone, N.J. (2000) The Gruppo Italiano per lo Studio della Sopravvivenza nell'Infarto Miocardio (GISSI)-Prevenzione Trial on fish oil and vitamin E supplementation in myocardial infarction survivors. *Curr. Cardiol. Rep.*, **2**, 445-51.

Southon, S. (2000) Increased fruit and vegetable consumption within the EU: potential health benefits. *Food Res. Int.*, **33**, 211-17.

Tunstall-Pedoe, H., Kuulasmaa, K., Mahonen, M., Tolonen, H., Ruokokaski, E. & Amouyel, P. (1999) Contribution in survival and coronary-event rates to changes in coronary heart disease mortality: 10-year results from 37 WHO MONICA Project populations. *Lancet*, **353**, 1547-57.

van den Berg, H., Faulks, R., Granado, H.F., Hirchberg, J., Olmedilla, B., Sandmann, G., Southon, S. & Stahl, W. (2000) The potential for the improvement of carotenoid levels in foods and likely systemic effects. *J. Sci. Food Agric.*, **80**, 880-912.

3

A BRIEF REVIEW OF THE IMPACT OF DIETARY POLYPHENOLS ON CARDIOVASCULAR DISEASE

GARY WILLIAMSON

Why polyphenols?

Polyphenols are found in most plant foods, but especially in wine, onions, tea, broccoli, cocoa products and apples and many other fruits. There is considerable epidemiological and mechanistic data to show that diets high in polyphenols protect against chronic diseases such as cardio-vascular disease. However, *in vivo* data using suitable biomarkers of effect are not available to assess the real impact of polyphenols on health. Many studies on flavonoid bioavailability are not of a suitable quality to assess uptake and metabolism of polyphenols. This chapter reviews briefly the epidemiological evidence for a protective effect, together with informa-tion from selected papers on the biological activities that could give rise to a protection. This chapter is not intended for experts in polyphenols, but as an introduction for dietitians and nutritionists who are familiar with nutrients but have yet to be introduced to the complex area of dietary polyphenols.

Classes of polyphenols

Unlike the vitamins, the chemical structures of polyphenols are extremely complex, and many classes and compounds are present in food. Adding together all of the polyphenols consumed in the diet from foods and beverages, the daily intake is probably in the region of a gram per day.

Polyphenols are derived solely from plants, and the total intake will be highly variable between individuals. Polyphenols are often divided into the classes shown in Figure 3.1. This is not an exhaustive list of all groups of polyphenols, only the most common dietary examples. Chemical structures can be found in many reviews (Pierpoint, 1986; Okuda *et al.*, 1995; Haslam, 1996; Bravo, 1998; Clifford, 1999). There are numerous reviews on the polyphenol contents of foods (Herrmann, 1976, 1989).

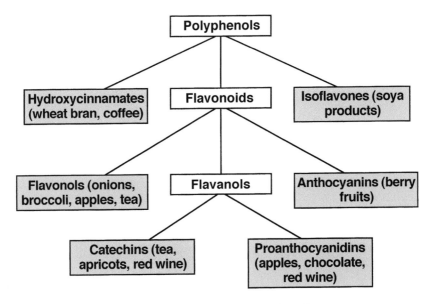

Figure 3.1　Relationship between classes of polyphenols.

Contents of polyphenols in foods

Table 3.1 shows the typical polyphenol content of some foods that are commonly consumed. Onions, especially red onions, apples and black tea are particularly high in flavonols, e.g. quercetin. This compound has been studied extensively, although most have focused on the aglycone form because it can be purchased but this form is almost non-existent in foods. In foods, quercetin is found attached to a sugar moiety, which dramatically affects its properties. However, this glycoside form is either not available commercially or is very expensive. Researchers have taken the easy option and used the readily available aglycone form, even though it is unstable in physiological conditions (Boulton *et al.*, 2000). This illustrates one of the problems with this area of research.

Table 3.1 Approximate guideline values for some polyphenols in commonly-consumed foods. Values are in mg per 100 g or 200 ml for foods and beverages respectively.

	Flavonols	Catechin monomers	Proanthocyanidins
Tomato	0.5	—	—
Lettuce	1	—	—
Onion	36	—	—
Apple	4	11	100
Cherry	2	6	70
Dark chocolate	—	80	430
Red wine	3	50	70
Black tea	8	130	—

Only recently have data become available on the bioavailability of polyphenols such as quercetin, and it is still largely incomplete (Hollman & Katan, 1997a, 1997b; de Vries *et al.*, 1998; Hollman *et al.*, 2000; Scalbert & Williamson, 2000). It is clear that the chemical structure of polyphenols is modified, often substantially, during metabolism in the body. There is a huge body of evidence for biological activities of the aglycone form of quercetin for example, but this form is not found in significant amounts *in vivo*. Furthermore, the biological activities of the metabolites are largely unknown, except in a few cases (Manach *et al.*, 1998; Day *et al.*, 2000). This is a serious consideration when assessing the possible biological activities of polyphenols.

Epidemiology for reduced risk of cardiovascular disease

The epidemiological evidence for a protective effect of dietary polyphenol consumption against cardiovascular disease is mixed, although the majority of studies show a protective effect (Table 3.2). A recent example is illustrated by a prospective study using 34 492 post-menopausal women in Iowa, USA, with a 10 year follow-up involving 438 deaths from coronary heart disease and 131 deaths from stroke (Yochum *et al.*, 1999). In this study, total flavonoid intake was correlated with a decreased risk of cardiovascular disease-related death ($p = 0.04$), and broccoli was most associated with this effect. There was no relationship between flavonoid intake and risk of stroke mortality. The methodology used was a food frequency questionnaire using already-published flavonoid contents of foods. However, given the complexity and variability of the type and amount of polyphenols in foods, it is difficult to ensure that polyphenol consumption from questionnaires is accurate.

Table 3.2 Summary of the epidemiological evidence for effect of polyphenols on cardiovascular disease (Reviewed in Day & Williamson, 1999).

Study	Number in study	Age (years)	Relative risk of mortality from coronary heart disease[a]
Zutphen (The Netherlands)	805	65–84	0.32 (0.15–0.71)[b]
			0.47 (0.27–0.82)[c]
Finland	5133	30–69	0.73 (0.41–1.32)[d]
			0.67 (0.44–1.00)[e]
US male health professional	34789	40–75	1.31 (0.42–3.05)[f]
Caerphilly (Wales)	1900	49–59	1.6 (0.9–2.9)
Zutphen (The Netherlands)	552	50–69	0.27 (0.11–0.7)[g]

[a] after adjustment of known risk factors, [b] 5-year follow-up, [c] 10-year follow up, [d] female, [e] male, [f] prevalent CHD at baseline gives a relative risk of mortality of 0.63 (0.33–1.2), [g] incidence of stroke.

Mechanism of protection against cardiovascular disease

A biomarker is a short-term biochemical change indicating long-term protection (actually a reduction in risk) against a disease, in this case cardiovascular disease. A much-used biomarker is the protection of plasma low density lipoprotein (LDL) from oxidation. Oxidation of LDL is a difficult parameter to measure, as isolation of the LDL fraction from blood itself can cause oxidation. Two recent comparable studies reached opposing conclusions. *Ex vivo* oxidisability of plasma LDL was measured after black tea consumption (6 cups per day). In one study, there was a 15% increase in lag time (i.e. protection) for Cu^{2+}-induced oxidation of LDL ($n = 22$, 5 cups Twinings Darjeeling (11 g dry weight) per day for 4 weeks) (Ishikawa *et al.*, 1997). In the second study, there was no change in lag time for Cu^{2+}-induced oxidation of LDL ($n = 32$, 6 cups Liptons tea (18 g dry weight) per day for 4 weeks) (van het Hof *et al.*, 1997). There were no changes in LDL lipid composition in either study. One problem with many studies of this type is that the dietary intervention is short or medium term: in the above studies, it was for 4 weeks, but for many it is often just one meal or beverage (Boyle *et al.*, 2000). In reality, dietary benefits of food are probably accrued over many years or even decades, but current funding strategies of granting agencies do not facilitate this sort of study. Addition of milk would not be expected to greatly affect the biological activities of tea polyphenols, and indeed a study has shown this (van het Hof *et al.*, 1998).

Further studies have addressed polyphenols from sources other than tea. Dietary intakes of flavonoids and isoflavones were associated with a lower level of plasma total cholesterol and LDL-cholesterol in 115 Japanese women aged 29–78 (Arai *et al.*, 2000). The best correlation for a single component was for the polyphenol quercetin. Onions were the major source of flavonols, whereas tofu was the major source of isoflavones. The possible mechanism of protection of LDL by quercetin has been studied by many authors. The aglycone (i.e. free) quercetin inhibits copper-induced peroxidation of LDL with TBARS detection with IC_{50} of 0.22 µM (Vinson *et al.*, 1995), and quercetin inhibited Cu^{2+}-induced LDL oxidation: 1 µM prolonged lag phase by ~3-fold (Brown *et al.*, 1998). These studies show that quercetin is a more potent inhibitor of human LDL oxidation than flavanols such as catechin. However, a recent study showed that quercetin from onions (1 dose of 225 g) fed to five healthy volunteers altered plasma antioxidant capacity but not LDL susceptibility, but only a single dose was given (Boyle *et al.*, 2000).

However, an important point which has been missed by most studies is that quercetin is metabolised during passage through the small intestine and subsequently by the liver to conjugates, and these conjugates with glucuronic acid, sulfates, methyl groups or glycine are the only circulating forms of quercetin. Identification of quercetin glycosides in plasma is probably as a result of misidentification (Day & Williamson, 1999). The conjugate can have very different, or comparable, biological activities compared to the aglycone depending on the position of substitution of the glucuronic acid (Day *et al.*, 2000). There is also very limited information on the long term effects of quercetin or other polyphenol consumption on LDL oxidisability.

It is clear that there are many gaps in our knowledge on the effect of polyphenols on human health. Even for well-studied vitamins and minerals, the links between doses above subsistence level and chronic disease are notoriously difficult to prove. This difficulty leads to problems with health claims on food products. With the predicted increase in the functional food market in the twenty-first century, ensuring that the consumer is not misled but has access to the most healthy foods, is a major challenge in the future.

Acknowledgements

The work carried out at the Institute of Food Research and described in this article was funded predominantly by the Biotechnology and Biological Sciences Research Council, UK, and the European Union (QLK1-1999-00505).

References

Arai, Y., Watanabe, S., Kimira, M., Shimoi, K., Mochizuki, R. & Kinae, N. (2000) Dietary intakes of flavonols, flavones and isoflavones by Japanese women and the inverse correlation between quercetin intake and plasma LDL cholesterol concentration. *J.Nutr.*, **130**, 2243-50.

Boulton, D.W., Walle, K. & Walle, T. (2000) Fate of the flavonoid quercetin in human cell lines; chemical instability and metabolism. *J.Pharm.Pharmacol.*, **51**, 353-9.

Boyle, S.P., Dobson,V.L., Duthie, S.J., Kyle, J.A.M. & Collins, A.R. (2000) Absorption and DNA protective effects of flavonoid glycosides from an onion meal. *Eur.J.Nutr.*, **39**, 213-23.

Bravo, L. (1998) Polyphenols: Chemistry, dietary sources, metabolism, and nutritional significance. *Nutr.Rev.*, **56**, 317-33.

Brown, J., Khodr, H., Hider, R.C. & Rice-Evans, C. (1998) Structural dependence of flavonoid interactions with Cu^{2+} ions: implications for their antioxidant properties. *Biochem.J.*, **330**, 1173-8.

Clifford, M.N. (1999) The nature of chlorogenic acids – are they advantageous compounds in coffee? *J.Sci.Food Agric.*, **79**, 1-13.

Day, A.J., Bao,Y.P., Morgan, M.R.A. & Williamson, G. (2000) Conjugation position of quercetin glucuronides and effect on biological activity. *Free Rad.Biol.Med.*, **29**, 1234-43.

Day, A.J. & Williamson, G. (1999) Metabolism of dietary quercetin glycosides by humans. In: *Plant polyphenols 2: Chemistry, Biology, Pharmacology and Ecology* (eds Gross, G.G., Hemingway, R.W., Yoshida, T.), pp 415-34, Kluwer Academic/Plenum, New York.

de Vries, J.H.M., Hollman, P.C.H., Meyboom, S., Buysman, M.N.C.P., Zock, P.L., van Staveren, W.A. & Katan, M.B. (1998) Plasma concentrations and urinary excretion of the antioxidant flavonols quercetin and kaempferol as biomarkers for dietary intake. *Am.J.Clin. Nutr.*, **68**, 60-65.

Haslam, E. (1996) Natural polyphenols (vegetable tannins) as drugs: Possible modes of action. *J.Nat.Prod.Lloydia.*, **59**, 205-15.

Herrmann, K. (1976) Flavanols and flavones in food plants: a review. *J.Food Technol.*, **11**, 433-48.

Herrmann, K. (1989) Occurrence and content of hydroxycinnamic and hydroxybenzoic acid compounds in foods. *Crit.Rev.Sci.Nutrition*, **28**, 315-47.

Hollman, P.C.H., Bijsman, M.N.C.P., van Gameren,Y., Cnossen, E.P.J., de Vries, J.H.M. & Katan, M.B. (2000) The sugar moiety is a major determinant of the absorption of dietary flavonoid glycosides in man. *Free Rad.Res.*, **31**, 569-73.

Hollman, P.C.H. & Katan, M.B. (1997a) Absorption, metabolism and health effects of dietary flavonoids in man. *Biomed.Pharmacother.*, **51**, 305-10.

Hollman, P.C.H., van Trijp, J.M.P., Mengelers, M.J.B., deVries, J.H.M. & Katan, M.B. (1997b) Bioavailability of the dietary antioxidant flavonol quercetin in man. *Cancer Lett.*, **114**, 139-40.

Ishikawa, T., Suzukawa, M., Ito, T., Yoshida, H., Ayaori, M., Nishiwaki, M., Yonemura, A., Hara,Y. & Nakamura, H. (1997) Effect of tea flavonoid supplementation on the susceptibility of low-density lipoprotein to oxidative modification. *Am.J.Clin.Nutr.*, **66**, 261-6.

Manach, C., Morand, C., Crespy, V., Demigne, C., Texier, O., Regerat, F. &

Remesy, C. (1998) Quercetin is recovered in human plasma as conjugated derivatives which retain antioxidant properties. *FEBS lett.*, **426**, 331-6.

Okuda, T., Yoshida, T. & Hatano, T. (1995) Hydrolyzable tannins and related polyphenols. *Prog.Chem.Org.Nat.Prod.*, **66**, 1-117.

Pierpoint, W.S. (1986) Flavonoids in the human diet. In: *Plant Flavonoids in the Human Diet: Biochemical, Pharmacological and Structure-activity Relationships* (eds Cody,V., Middleton, E. Jr. & Harborne, J.B.), pp. 125-40, A.R. Liss, New York.

Scalbert, A. & Williamson, G. (2000) Dietary intake and bioavailability of polyphenols. *J.Nutr.*, **130**, 2073S-2085S.

van het Hof, K.H., de Boer, H.S.M., Wiseman, S.A., Lien, N., Weststrate, J.A. & Tijburg, L.B.M. (1997) Consumption of green or black tea does not increase resistance of low-density lipoprotein to oxidation in humans. *Am.J.Clin.Nutr.*, **66**, 1125-32.

van het Hof, K.H., Kivits, G.A.A., Weststrate, J.A. & Tijburg, L.B.M. (1998) Bioavailability of catechins from tea: the effect of milk. *Eur.J.Clin.Nutr.*, **52**, 356-9.

Vinson, J.A., Dabbagh, Y.A., Serry, M.M. & Jang, J.H. (1995) Plant flavonoids, especially tea flavonols, are powerful antioxidants using an in vitro oxidation model for heart disease. *J.Agr.Food Chem.*, **43**, 2800-802.

Yochum, L., Kushi, L.H., Meyer, K. & Folsom, A.R. (1999) Dietary flavonoid intake and risk of cardiovascular disease in post-menopausal women. *Am.J.Epidemiol.*, **149**, 943-9.

4

SIGNIFICANCE OF CHOLESTEROL ABSORPTION: INHIBITORY ROLE OF PLANT STEROLS AND STANOLS

GILBERT R. THOMPSON

Recent research suggests that net absorption of cholesterol reflects both intestinal uptake via a saturable pathway and ABC 1-mediated efflux. Genetically-determined variability in absorption underlies hypo- and hyper-responsiveness of plasma LDL-cholesterol to dietary cholesterol. Inhibiting uptake of cholesterol by pharmacological agents or by consumption of plant sterol and stanol esters provides an effective and safe means of lowering LDL. The extent of reduction can be enhanced by combining these approaches with concomitant statin therapy.

Cholesterol is an essential constituent of mammalian cell membranes and is also present in plasma. The main sources of cholesterol in the body are from *de novo* synthesis via the HMG CoA reductase pathway, especially in the liver, adrenals and gonads, and absorption of dietary cholesterol in the small intestine. Depending upon the dietary intake, approximately 1 g of cholesterol enters the duodenum every 24 hours, two-thirds of which is of biliary origin. This mixes with dietary cholesterol in the intestinal lumen to form a single pool, roughly 50% of which undergoes absorption during its passage through the jejunum. There is considerable interindividual variation in the efficiency of cholesterol absorption and this is reflected in the concentration of LDL-cholesterol in plasma, which, in turn, is a major determinant of the risk of developing coronary heart disease (CHD). Consequently, there is increasing interest in dietetic and pharmacological approaches to lowering LDL-cholesterol by inhibiting cholesterol absorption.

Absorptive mechanisms

The process whereby cholesterol is solubilised within the intestinal lumen by incorporation into mixed micelles is well described. These particles consist mainly of bile salts and the end products of pancreatic lipolysis of dietary triglyceride, namely free fatty acids and monoglycerides. However, the subsequent steps whereby cholesterol is selectively taken up by the brush border membrane and transported through the enterocyte have hitherto been poorly understood, apart from the fact that intestinal acylCoA:cholesterol:acyl transferase (ACAT) is known to esterify cholesterol prior to its incorporation into chylomicrons and secretion into intestinal lymph.

Recently, a specific and saturable pathway has been identified which mediates the transport of cholesterol from mixed micelles into enterocytes (Hernandez *et al.*, 2000; Detmers *et al.*, 2000). If confirmed this discovery of the cholesterol transporter will greatly enhance our understanding of how cholesterol absorption is regulated. Another recent and equally important advance is the discovery of the role of the ATP-binding cassette transporter (ABC 1) in the reverse transport of cholesterol from cells, including the small intestine (McNeish *et al.*, 2000). Reverse transport of cholesterol is lacking in ABC 1 knock-out mice, an animal model of Tangier disease, whereas upregulation of this pathway in intact animals promotes intestinal efflux of cholesterol and thereby limits the net amount absorbed (Repa *et al.*, 2000).

Influence of cholesterol absorption on plasma cholesterol

An association between the efficiency with which cholesterol is absorbed and the concentration of cholesterol in plasma, especially in LDL, has long been recognised. In part, this derives from observations in both experimental animals and man concerning the basis of the twin phenomena of hypo- and hyper-responsiveness to dietary cholesterol. It has been shown that hypo-responders absorb a lower percentage of cholesterol than do hyper-responders when the dietary intake is raised and exhibit a smaller increase in LDL-cholesterol. As discussed elsewhere, the likelihood is that these traits are genetically determined (Thompson, in press). For example, possession of the apoE$_4$ allele appears to be associated with a hyper-absorptive and hyper-responsive tendency. In normal subjects the efficiency with which cholesterol is absorbed decreases when the intake is raised (Ostlund *et al.*, 1999) and it seems that hyper-responders lack this adaptive response. Apart from apoE genotype, another putative source of genetic variation in regulating net cholesterol absorption is the ABC 1 gene, which has recently been sequenced (Santamarina-Fojo *et al.*, 2000).

Evidence that cholesterol absorption efficiency and LDL-cholesterol concentration are causally related comes from studies of pharmacological inhibitors of cholesterol absorption. For example, it has long been known that neomycin, a polycationic antibiotic, interacts with bile acid and fatty acid anions to precipitate mixed micelles and thereby inhibits cholesterol absorption (Thompson *et al.*, 1971). More recent studies have shown a linear correlation between inhibition of cholesterol absorption and reduction in LDL-cholesterol in subjects given neomycin (Gylling & Miettinen, 1995). Furthermore, the novel compound ezetimibe, which inhibits absorption of cholesterol by a different mechanism, lowers LDL-cholesterol also and in a dose-related manner (Bays *et al.*, 2000).

Role of plant sterols and stanols

It has long been known that plant sterols inhibit the absorption of cholesterol, with which they are closely related structurally, and more recently plant stanols have been shown to do the same. Plant sterols occur naturally in vegetable oils, such as soybean and rapeseed, whereas plant stanols are found in tall oil, a side product of the manufacture of paper from conifers. The main plant sterols, sitosterol and campesterol, are readily converted to their stanol counterparts, sitostanol and campestanol, by hydrogenation.

Initially, when they were administered as free sterols and stanols, the latter appeared to be more effective in inhibiting cholesterol absorption and lowering LDL-cholesterol. This superiority was most marked with sitostanol, the predominant stanol in tall oil, which is virtually unabsorbed when ingested, whereas campestanol, sitosterol and especially campesterol are all absorbed to some extent. All these compounds compete with cholesterol for incorporation into mixed micelles, with sitostanol the most effective in this respect. However, the limited lipid solubility of free sterols and stanols makes them difficult to incorporate into spreads in high enough concentrations to be effective. This limitation was subsequently overcome by esterifying these compounds with long chain fatty acids, which increased their lipid solubility and thus facilitated their incorporation into foods. Hence, any evaluation of currently marketed products should be based on studies involving esterified rather than free sterols and stanols.

To date three direct comparisons of the efficacy and safety of plant sterol and stanol esters have been published (Weststrate & Meijer, 1998; Hallikainen *et al.*, 2000; Jones *et al.*, 2000), details of which are shown in Table 4.1. Daily consumption, expressed as free sterol or stanol, ranged from 1.8 to 3.1 g daily for periods of 3–4 weeks each. As shown in Figure 4.1, the LDL-lowering efficacy of plant sterol and stanol esters were similar, with weighted means of -12.4% and -11.7% respectively. The main difference between the two compounds was that the plasma levels of campesterol and sitosterol, expressed as ratios to total cholesterol, increased on plant sterols but fell on plant stanols (Table 4.2). It remains to be shown whether this difference is of any clinical significance other than in patients with the rare disorder phytosterolaemia, which is characterised by excessive absorption of plant sterols, resulting in markedly elevated plasma sitosterol and campesterol levels and premature atherosclerosis. Administration of plant sterol esters is contraindicated in such circumstances whereas plant stanol esters could be beneficial.

Table 4.1 Comparative studies of plant sterol and stanol esters at equivalent intakes.

Study	Subjects			Diet		Dose g/d		Duration
	Type	n	Age (years)	Fat, g	Chol, mg	Sterol	Stanol	
Westrate & Meijer, 1998	NC/HC	95	45	32	230	3.1	2.7	3 weeks
Jones *et al.*, 2000	HC	15	37–61	35	not measured	1.8	1.8	3 weeks
Hallikainen *et al.*	HC	34	49	30	175	2.0	2.0	4 weeks

NC = normocholesterolaemic; HC = hypercholesterolaemic

The comparable LDL-lowering ability of equivalent amounts of plant sterol and stanol esters reflects the fact that they induce almost identical decreases in cholesterol absorption and compensatory increases in cholesterol synthesis (Normen *et al.*, 2000). In addition, Plat and Mensink (2000) have shown that wood-derived (i.e. sitostanol-rich) and vegetable oil-derived (i.e. campestanol-rich) stanol esters had similar LDL-lowering properties. These authors have also made the important observation that

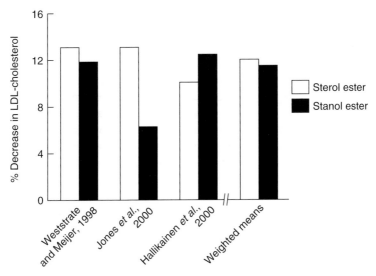

Figure 4.1 Efficacy of plant sterol and stanol esters in three comparative trials (see Table 4.1).

Table 4.2 Changes in plasma plant sterols in subjects consuming sterol and stanol esters.

Diet	Study	Change in plasma ratio v control	
		Campesterol/TC	Sitosterol/TC
Sterol ester	Westrate & Meijer, 1998	89%	52%
	Jones *et al.*, 2000	93%	39%
	Hallikainen *et al.*, 2000	47%	34%
Stanol ester	Westrate & Meijer, 1998	− 11%	− 33%
	Jones *et al.*, 2000	− 12%	− 10%
	Hallikainen *et al.*, 2000	− 28%	− 30%

TC = total cholesterol

single and divided doses of equivalent amounts of plant stanol ester have similar LDL-lowering effects (Plat *et al.*, 2000). In contrast, plasma levels of α plus β carotene plus lycopene were significantly reduced after the divided dose regimen but not after single daily doses of plant stanol. These findings suggest that micellar competition is not the sole mechanism whereby cholesterol absorption is inhibited, in contrast to carotene, and suggests that, in addition, stanols have a prolonged residence in the intestinal mucosa, as was shown to occur with plant sterols more than 40 years ago (Swell *et al.*, 1959).

The potential cardiovascular benefits of lowering LDL-cholesterol in the population at large by daily consumption of plant sterol and stanol esters have been discussed by Law (2000). In addition, there is evidence that plant stanol esters enhance the LDL-lowering effects of statins when given concomitantly to moderately hypercholesterolaemic individuals (Blair *et al.*, 2000), to patients with familial hypercholesterolaemia (Vuorio *et al.*, 2000) and in the secondary prevention of coronary heart disease (Gylling *et al.*, 1997). Thus, the introduction of stanol ester-containing products has provided a new dimension to the dietary management of dyslipidaemia by enabling 10–15% reductions in LDL-cholesterol to be achieved safely on a long-term basis (Miettinen *et al.*, 1995).

References

Bays, H., Drehobl, M., Rosenblatt, S., Toth, P., Dujovne, C., Knopp, R., Lipka, L., Cuffie-Jackson, C. (2000) Low-density lipoprotein cholesterol reduction by SCH 58235 (ezetimibe), a novel inhibitor of intestinal cholesterol absorption in 243 hypercholesterolemic subjects: Results of a dose-response study. *Atherosclerosis*, **151**, 135.

Blair, S.N., Capuzzi, D.M., Gottlieb, S.O., Nguyen, T., Morgan, J.M. & Cater, N.B. (2000) Incremental reduction of serum total cholesterol and low-density lipoprotein cholesterol with the addition of plant stanol ester-containing spread to statin therapy. *Am. J. Cardiol.*, **86**, 46–52.

Detmers, P.A., Patel, S., Hernandez, M., Montenegro, J., Lisnock, J.M., Pikounis, B. Steiner, M., Kim, D., Sparrow, C., Chao, Y.S. & Wright, S.D. (2000) A target for cholesterol absorption inhibitors in the enterocyte brush border membrane. *Biochim. Biophys. Acta.*, **19**, 243–52.

Gylling, H., Radhakrishnan, R. & Miettinen, T.A. (1997) Reduction of serum cholesterol in postmenopausal women with previous myocardial infarction and cholesterol malabsorption induced by dietary sitostanol ester margarine: women and dietary sitostanol. *Circulation*, **96**, 4226–31.

Gylling, H. & Miettinen, T.A. (1995) The effect of cholesterol absorption inhibition on low density lipoprotein cholesterol level. *Atherosclerosis*, **117**, 305–8.

Hallikainen, M.A., Sarkinnen, E.S., Gylling, H., Erkilla, A.T., & Uusitupa, M.J.J. (2000) Comparison of the effects of plant sterol ester and plant stanol ester-enriched margarines in lowering serum cholesterol concentrations in hypercholesterolaemic subjects on a low-fat diet. *Eur. J. Clin. Nutr.*, **54**, 715–25.

Hernandez, M., Montenegro, J., Steiner, M., Kim, D., Sparrow, C., Detmers, P.A., Wright, S.D. & Chao, Y.S. (2000) Intestinal absorption of cholesterol is mediated by a saturable, inhibitable transporter. *Biochim. Biophys. Acta.*, **19**, 232–42.

Jones, P.J., Raeini-Sarjaz, M., Ntanios, F.Y., Vanstone, C.A., Feng, J.Y. & Parsons, W.E. (2000) Modulation of plasma lipid levels and cholesterol kinetics by phytosterol versus phytostanol esters. *J. Lipid Res.*, **41**, 697-705.

Law, M. (2000) Plant sterol and stanol margarines and health. *BMJ*, **320**, 861–4.

McNeish, J., Aiello, R.J., Guyot, D., Turi, T., Gabel, C., Aldinger, C., Hoppe, K.L.,

Roach, M.L., Royer, L.J., de Wet, J., Broccardo, C., Chimini, G. & Francone, O.L. (2000) High density lipoprotein deficiency and foam cell accumulation in mice with targeted disruption of ATP-binding cassette transporter-1. *Proc. Natl. Acad. Sci., USA*, **97**, 4245–50.

Miettinen, T.A., Puska, P., Gylling, H., Vanhanen, H. & Vartiainen, E. (1995) Reduction of serum cholesterol with sitostanol-ester margarine in a mildly hypercholesterolemic population. *N. Engl. J. Med.*, **333**, 1308–12.

Normen, L., Dutta, P., Lia, A. & Andersson, H. (2000) Soy sterol esters and β-sitostanol ester as inhibitors of cholesterol absorption in human small bowel. *Am. J. Clin. Nutr.*, **71**, 908–13.

Ostlund, R.E., Bosner, M.S. Jr., Stenson, W.F. (1999) Cholesterol absorption efficiency declines at moderate dietary doses in normal human subjects. *J. Lipid Res.*, **40**, 1453–8.

Plat, J. & Mensink, R.P. (2000) Vegetable oil based versus wood based stanol ester mixtures: effects on serum lipids and hemostatic factors in non-hypercholesterolemic subjects. *Atherosclerosis*, **148**, 101–12.

Plat, J., Van Onselen, E.N.M., van Heugten, M.M. & Mensink, R.P. (2000) Effects on serum lipids, lipoproteins and fat soluble antioxidant concentrations of consumption frequency of margarines and shortenings enriched with plant stanol esters. *Eur. J. Clin. Nutr.*, **54**, 671–7.

Repa, J.J., Turley, S.D., Lobaccaro, J.A., Medina, J., Li, L., Lustig, K., Shan, B., Heyman, R.A., Dietschy, J.M. & Mangelsdorf, D.J. (2000) Regulation of absorption and ABC1-mediated efflux of cholesterol by RXR heterodimers. *Science*, **289**, 1524–9.

Santamarina-Fojo, S., Peterson, K., Knapper, C., Qiu, Y., Freeman, L., Cheng, J.F., Osorio, J., Remaley, A., Yang, X.P., Haudenschild, C., Prades, C., Chimini, G., Blackmon, E., Francois, T., Duverger, N., Rubin, E.M., Rosier, M.. Denefle, P., Fredrickson, D.S. & Brewer, H.B. Jr. (2000) Complete genomic sequence of the human ABCA1 gene: analysis of the human and mouse ATP-binding cassette A promoter. *Proc. Natl Acad. Sci. USA*, **97**, 7987–92.

Swell, L., Trout, E.C. Jr., Field, H. Jr. & Treadwell, C.R. (1959) Intestinal metabolism of C14-phytosterols. *J. Biol. Chem.*, **234**, 2286.

Thompson, G.R. (in press) Genetic influence on cholesterol absorption and its therapeutic consequences.

Thompson, G.R., Barrowman, J., Gutierrez, L. & Dowling, R.H. (1971) Action of neomycin on the intraluminal phase of lipid absorption. *J. Clin. Invest.*, **50**, 319–23.

Vuorio, A.F., Gylling, H., Turtola, H., Kontula, K., Ketonen, P. & Miettinen, T.A. (2000) Stanol ester margarine alone and with simvastatin lowers serum cholesterol in families with familial hypercholesterolaemia caused by the FH-North Karelia mutation. *Arterioscler. Thromb. Vasc. Biol.*, **20**, 500–506.

Weststrate, J.A. & Meijer, G.W. (1998) Plant sterol-enriched margarines and reduction of plasma total- and LDL-cholesterol concentrations in normocholesterolaemic and mildly hypercholesterolaemic subjects. *Eur. J. Clin. Nutr.*, **52**, 334–43.

5

SOYA AND THE FDA HEALTH CLAIM: PREVENTION OF CARDIOVASCULAR DISEASES

JAAK PH. JANSSENS

Cardiovascular diseases (CVD), particularly coronary heart diseases (CHD), are responsible for the largest number of hospitalisations in Western countries and consume by far the highest part of the health care budget (Bendich & Deckelbaum, 1997). It can be estimated that half of the costs of the health care budget for CVD, risk of disease and mortality can be effectively reduced by prevention. In this overview, the power of prevention by nutrition is gauged as well as the contribution of soy derivatives to this prevention. Finally, the Food and Drug Administration's (FDA) food labelling health claim on soy protein and CHD is discussed.

Risk factors for CVD and prevention through nutrition

Male gender, age, smoking, hypertension, obesity, diabetes and cholesterol are the best known risk factors for atherosclerosis and CVD (see Table 5.1). Many of these factors are causal and can be managed by lifestyle and diet. Not smoking, the lowering of LDL-cholesterol in the blood, Mediterranean food, physical exercise and control of hypertension are well established and most of them work through the lowering of serum cholesterol. In fact, there is an almost linear to exponential correlation between serum cholesterol and risk of and mortality from CVD. Based on this simple relation, nutritional and lifestyle measures to lower serum cholesterol are encouraged in all Western countries for the whole popu-

Table 5.1 Cardiovascular disease risk factors.

Demography	Age
	Male gender
	Menopausal status
Lifestyle	Smoking
	Physical activity
	Obesity
Medical	Hypertension
	Diabetes
	Hyperhomocystinemia
Lipid disorders	Hypercholesterolemia
	Increase in LDL-cholesterol
	Decrease in HDL-cholesterol
	Hypertriglycidemia
	Increases in apolipoprotein B
	Decreases in apolipoprotein A1
	Increase in oxidized LDL-cholesterol
	Increase of small dens LDL-cholesterol
	Increase in lipoproteins
	Apolipoprotein E4 allele
Haemostasis	Increase in fibrinogen
	Increase in factor VII
	Increase in von Willebrand factor
	Increase in Plasminogen activator inhibitor
Infections	Cytomegalovirus
	Chlamydia pneumoniae
	Helicobacter pylori
Inflammation	White blood cell count
	C-reactive protein
	Serum amyloid protein
	Intercellular adhesion molecule-1

lation. In addition, consensus emerges that these dietary measures should have a priority in the treatment of moderate hypercholesterolemia (>190 mg%).

Cholesterol is transported in the blood through the solvent properties of high (HDL) and low density lipoproteins (LDL). About 70% of the cholesterol is bound to LDL. A high amount of cholesterol bound to the LDL group is correlated with increased risk of CVD of which CHDs are the most common. Increased binding to HDL lowers the risk. Higher trigly-

ceride levels increase the risk of CVD as well. Nutrition can alter the lipoprotein profile of the blood. Lowering dietary cholesterol (C) lowers plasma cholesterol and LDL-C in humans depending on the expression of the apoprotein isoforms and decreases the risk of CVD. Also the lipoprotein status of the host, affected both by previous and concurrent dietary or longstanding genetic factors, dictates the potential impact on cholesterol rise after intake of high cholesterol foods and saturated fat.

An increased intake in short and middle chain saturated fatty acids (SFAs >C12) increases the LDL and to a lesser extent HDL fractions. Increased consumption of stearine FA (C18) has a similar effect to carbohydrates and increases LDL and HDL-type cholesterol. Palmitine FA has an ambivalent effect on cholesterol. SFAs in general should be lowered in the diet from an average of 14% to about 10% of total energy intake. Mono-unsaturated FAs (MUFAs) are recently getting more attention because they do not increase triacylglycerol and lower HDL. In addition, they seem to play a direct role in the inflammatory reaction at the initial steps of atherosclerosis (Massaro *et al.*, 1999). The polyunsaturated FAs (PUFAs) decrease LDL and increase HDL. The LDL response is non-linear with an apparent threshold at 5% of energy intake level.

The old dogma says that PUFAs should be increased in the diet. Probably the most favourable LDL/HDL ratio (i.e. lowest LDL and highest HDL) is induced by a diet with 30% energy as fat containing a combination of 16:0-rich SFAs (to elevate HDL) and PUFAs (to assure removal of LDL by the liver), each representing 8–10%. The intake of cholesterol can be modified also by inhibition of intestinal absorption through phytosterols and phytostanols. Oat bran diets containing glucan, a cholesterol binding water soluble gum, significantly increase faecal sterol elimination.

Non-oxidized LDL are recognised by receptors, which can be saturated, in contrast to oxidized LDL which cause an unlimited accumulation in the intima cells of arteries without the characteristics of saturation. The formation of the resulting 'foam cells' is a first sign of atherosclerosis. Endothelial damage is seen subsequently along with monocyte/macrophage recruitment, alteration in vascular tone and induction of growth factors. If this hypothesis is true, antioxidants may cause a significant reduction of atherosclerosis but up to now, the results of implementation trials are very disappointing. The polyphenols, which include the flavonoids, are worth studying because they are potent antioxidants and present in various foods.

Derived from methionine, homocysteine is an intermediary amino acid positively related to CVD. The evidence is very strong and consistent with an estimated risk of 1.6 for males and 1.5 for females for an increase of 5 μmol/L. Atherogenic mechanisms promoted by homocysteine include endothelial cell desquamation, oxidation of LDL and monocyte adhesion to the vessel wall. The concentration of homocysteine depends on genetic, lifestyle and nutritional factors and individuals with concentrations beyond 15 μmol/L are considered to suffer from hyperhomocyteinemia. Total homocysteine levels of 10 μmol/L are considered 'healthy' and a reduction of 5 μmol/L from 15 to 10 seems beneficial. Nutritional factors are folic acid, vitamin B12 and B6. Up to now, no study or randomised clinical trials firmly relate dietary folate intake or folic acid with the risk of CVD.

Soy protein metabolism

An increased consumption of soya products can provide a large amount of protein with a high amino acid quality and is associated with a very low incidence of cardiovascular disease. Serum and LDL-cholesterol concentrations can be lowered by approximately 13%. The plasma triglycerides are lowered by about 10% and the HDL is somewhat increased by 2%. The action of soya protein presumably is not at the intestinal level. Soya contains a heterogeneous mixture of proteins, the bulk being 7S and 11S globulins, and variable amounts of minor components, including isoflavones – consisting largely of genistein and daidzein – phytic acid and saponins. All these components can have a contribution to the LDL lowering effects of soya protein.

Studies in validated animal models and in humans have suggested that soya protein might directly activate LDL receptors in liver cells, which are chronically depressed in hypercholesterolemia. The responsible proteins include the 7S globulin, one of the major storage proteins of soya beans, and more precisely, the α and α' sub units. These proteins directly up-regulate LDL receptor expression by 50% or more. Soya protein, particularly the 7S globulin, lowers hepatic production of LDL structural protein, apo B, which is associated with a reduced rate of synthesis of cellular lipids, free cholesterol, cholesteryl esters and triacylglycerols. Some reports have also demonstrated that treatment with soya protein results in moderate reductions of serum triacylglycerols and small increases of HDL-cholesterol concentrations. Soya protein with higher levels of isoflavones might have more robust effects. Nevertheless, there is no evidence that purified soya isoflavones can improve plasma lipid concentrations.

Genistein might have more potent effects in tissues expressing ERβ, including arterial walls. Genistein appears equally effective compared to 17β estradiol in inhibiting atherogenesis. Soya protein isolate with isoflavones has been shown to lower diastolic blood pressure in women. The SPI improves vascular function by inhibition of coronary artery vascular constriction in response to acetylcholine (endothelium-dependent vascular response). This effect has not been seen with purified soya isoflavones. Isoflavones might inhibit platelet activation and aggregation and reduce the amount of serotonin in the platelets, all of which could contribute to a reduction in coronary vasospasm and thrombosis.

Soya treatment significantly inhibits LDL oxidation. Studies suggest that the isoflavones also have effects on smooth muscle cells which are involved in atherosclerosis promotion and progression. Genistein inhibits the migration and proliferation of smooth muscle cells in vivo.

Food and Drug Administration guideline on food labelling

The validity of lowering total cholesterol and LDL-C by soya derivatives is recently supported by the US FDA, approving a health claim about the role of soya protein in reducing the risk of CHD. On 26 October 1999 the FDA finalised a rule that authorises the use, on food labels and in food labelling of products under FDA jurisdiction, of the health claims concerning the association between soya protein and reduced risk of CHD (Federal Register Part 11, 1999): '*25 grams of soy protein a day, as part of a diet low in saturated fat and cholesterol, may reduce the risk of heart disease*'. This authorisation is based on numerous publications on the subject and high consistency between the publications, almost all proving beneficial effects. The goal to reach a sufficient daily consumption is achievable through the amazing transformation possibilities of soya bean into various food constituents.

Conclusion

When added to maintenance of a body mass index under 25, a good physical condition, a lowered fat intake < 30% of total energy with SFAs < 10% of total energy, and avoidance of foods rich in cholesterol, soya protein may reduce the risk of heart disease through various mechanisms. The epidemiological and laboratory evidence is sufficient for the FDA to endorse the statement on food labels that soya may effectively reduce the risk of CHD.

References

Bendich, A. & Deckelbaum, R.J. (eds) (1997) *Preventive Nutrition. The Comprehensive Guide for Health Professionals*. Humana Press, Totowa, New Jersey.

Federal Register Part II (1999) *21 CFR Part 101: Food labelling: Health Claims: Soy Protein and Coronary Hearth Disease: Final Rule, October 26 1999*. Department of Health and Human Services, Food and Drug Administration.

Massaro, M., Carluccio, M.A. & De Caterina, R. (1999) Direct vascular antiatherogenic effects of oleic acid: a clue to the cardioprotective effects of the Mediterranean diet. *Cardiologia*, 44, 507–13.

6

NUTRITIONAL DETERMINANTS OF PLASMA HOMOCYSTEINE: IMPLICATIONS FOR RISK OF CARDIOVASCULAR DISEASE

ANNE M. MOLLOY

Introduction

Cardiovascular disease (CVD) remains one of the major causes of morbidity and mortality in the developed world. Decades of research have established a number of major lifestyle and genetic factors associated with this disease; nevertheless, these classic risk factors still do not explain why many people develop CVD and others do not. Several emerging nutritional and lifestyle risk factors are currently being investigated. One factor in particular, the possible role of plasma homocysteine, has received a great deal of attention in the past ten years. The evidence linking elevated plasma homocysteine to various forms of vascular disease is based on a substantial body of epidemiological work including prospective and retrospective case-control studies and observations of disease progress in subjects with inborn errors affecting homocysteine metabolism. Many of these studies indicate that homocysteine is an independent risk factor for CVD with the level of risk graded across the entire normal plasma range.

The control of plasma homocysteine is largely dependent on the efficient functioning of three enzymes that all require vitamins. These are vitamin B_6, vitamin B_{12} and folate. The sensitivity of this relationship is such that

the plasma homocysteine concentration is considered to be a bio-marker of inadequate folate, vitamin B_{12} and to a lesser extent vitamin B_6 status. Intervention studies suggest that a large percentage of apparently normal subjects have plasma homocysteine levels that can be reduced by vitamin supplementation, with folic acid having the strongest effect, followed by vitamin B_{12}. However, it remains to be seen whether strategies to lower plasma homocysteine in the general population would have the effect of reducing the prevalence of CVD.

In the past decade there has been an astonishing increase in research publications on the subject of homocysteine. To a large extent, this explosion can be traced back to two lines of research. On the one hand, observations originating some 40 years ago indicated that abnormalities of methionine metabolism might lead to the development of coronary artery disease (Finkelstein, 2000). At that time, reports described patients with an inborn error in the enzyme cystathionine β-synthase (CBS) which catabolised homocysteine (Mudd *et al.*, 1964). These homocystinuric patients had massive elevations of homocysteine in plasma and urine. Among the subsequent clinical effects was a high risk for atherosclerosis and early thrombosis (Mudd *et al.*, 1985).

Since homocysteine arose from the essential amino acid, methionine, it was initially unclear whether elevated homocysteine or elevated methionine levels in the plasma were the toxic agent. However, within a few years a patient with a defect in vitamin B_{12} metabolism was described who had homocystinuria without elevated methionine but had developed atherosclerosis (Finkelstein, 2000). This prompted McCully (1969) to suggest that high plasma homocysteine levels caused premature atherosclerosis in these subjects and furthermore to propose that elevated plasma homocysteine levels (for whatever reason) might be a risk factor for the development of atherosclerosis.

The second factor contributing to this explosion was the description in the mid 1980s of new sensitive methods to measure blood total homocysteine concentrations (Refsum *et al.*, 1985; Ueland *et al.*, 1993). This methodology revitalised the area and paved the way for the type of epidemiological studies required to test McCully's hypothesis. Now, more than three decades after McCully, the association of this metabolite with various forms of vascular disease has been amply demonstrated and it is widely considered that moderately elevated plasma homocysteine represents an independent risk factor for CVD, of the order of that imposed by cholesterol.

Synthesis and metabolism of homocysteine

Homocysteine is an intermediate in the metabolism of the essential amino acid methionine. As can be seen from Figure 6.1, methionine has a major metabolic role outside of its involvement in protein synthesis. In the activated form of S-adenosylmethionine (SAM), it is the unique biological source of methyl groups for a wide range of methylation reactions. These methylations include the modification of proteins, lipids, DNA, neurotransmittors, etc., and are crucial to processes such as gene expression, cell signalling mechanisms and normal neurological function. Even the catabolism of excess methionine by the liver requires as a first step the synthesis of SAM and the removal of the methyl group to an appropriate acceptor molecule.

The de-methylated product in all these methylation reactions is S-adenosylhomocysteine (SAH), which is converted to homocysteine by the removal of adenosine. Homocysteine is a highly reactive, toxic molecule that has been shown in cell culture systems to be particularly damaging to endothelial cell function, coagulation mechanisms and vascular smooth muscles (Weir & Scott, 1998). Therefore, its level in cells and in the plasma must be kept within very narrow limits. Metabolism of homocysteine involves two alternative processes, recycling to methionine or catabolism.

Homocysteine is converted back to methionine by addition of a methyl group. This is a complex reaction, catalysed by the enzyme methionine synthase and requiring the action of two vitamins: folate as the co-substrate carrying the methyl group to be transferred and vitamin B_{12} as a cofactor of the enzyme. The reaction completes a cycle in which the carbon-sulphur skeleton of methionine is preserved and methyl groups are channelled through folate cofactors to be used for essential biological methylations. A second folate-related enzyme is also crucial to this process, i.e. methylenetetrahydrofolate reductase (MTHFR), which supplies the methyl group required by methionine synthase in the form of the folate cofactor 5-methyltetrahydrofolate. Homocysteine may also be remethylated by betaine methyltransferase, using betaine as the methyl donor. However, this vitamin-independent reaction is largely confined to the liver and kidney (McKeever *et al.*, 1991). The alternative metabolic fate for homocysteine is catabolism to cystathionine. This is achieved via cystathionine-β-synthase (CBS), an enzyme that requires vitamin B_6 as a cofactor. Thus the metabolism of homocysteine within the cell requires three vitamins – vitamin B_6, vitamin B_{12} and folate.

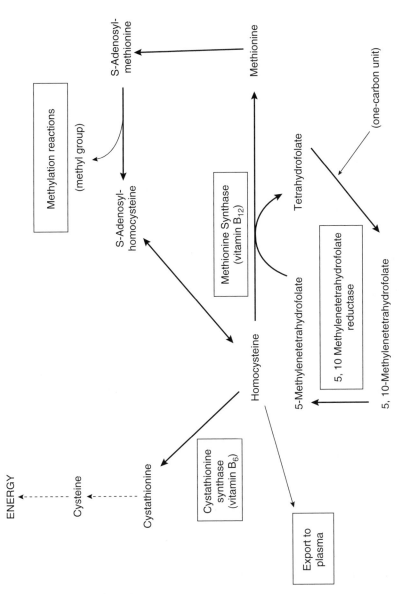

Figure 6.1 Pathways of homocysteine metabolism: Three key enzymes – methionine synthase, 5,10 methylenetetrahydrofolate reductase (MTHFR) and cystathionine β-synthase (CBS) are involved in this process. Methionine synthase uses a folate cofactor as co-substrate and vitamin B_{12} as a cofactor. MTHFR converts the folate cofactor to the required format for methionine synthase. CBS uses vitamin B_6 as a cofactor.

The level of homocysteine within cells and in the plasma is kept within very narrow limits by the efficient functioning of methionine synthase, MTHFR and CBS; however, this is dependent on an adequate nutrient intake. Even a modest reduction in the status of any of the three vitamins can disrupt the balance, causing an accumulation of intracellular SAH as well as increased export of homocysteine into the plasma (Ueland *et al.*, 1993). Indeed, it has been recognised for a decade that plasma homocysteine is a useful biochemical marker to detect early or subtle reduction in the status of folate, vitamin B_6 or vitamin B_{12} (Selhub *et al.*, 1993; Weir & Scott, 1998).

Most laboratories agree that the normal range for fasting plasma homocysteine is between 5 and 15 µmol/L; however, this is influenced by nutritional, genetic, medical and other factors (Ueland & Refsum, 1989; Eikelboom *et al.*, 1999; see Table 6.1). Of special interest in this regard is the recently identified common mutation in MTHFR (the C677T variant), which causes mild enzyme deficiency (Frosst *et al.*, 1995). This variant has a homozygous prevalence in various populations of 5% to 20%. These homozygous individuals tend to have moderately elevated plasma homocysteine levels (Frosst *et al.*, 1995). Another group of interest is the elderly. Hyperhomocysteinemia is frequently observed in this group and it has been suggested that elevated plasma homocysteine levels (>2 SD above the mean) may occur in up to 30% of apparently normal elderly individuals (Selhub *et al.*, 1993).

Table 6.1 Factors affecting the plasma homocysteine level.

General – Male sex, increasing age, menopause.
Nutritional – Deficiency/inadequate status of folate, vitamin B_{12}, vitamin B_6.
Diseases – Pernicious anaemia, renal disease, severe psoriasis, rheumatoid arthritis, hypothyroidism, some cancers.
Drugs and toxins – Folate antagonists (anticonvulsants, methotrexate), vitamin B_6 antagonists, oral contraceptives, cigarettes.
Genetic defects – CBS, MTHFR, methionine synthase and related vitamin B_{12} reducing enzymes.

Homocysteine and cardiovascular disease (CVD)

The evidence that homocysteine is a risk factor for CVD has been derived from a variety of sources including clinical observation of subjects with inborn errors of the three enzymes that control the plasma level of homocysteine, data from retrospective and prospective studies and correlation of homocysteine with disease progress and mortality. These lines of evidence have been reviewed in detail (Weir & Scott, 1998; Eikelboom *et al.*, 1999; Christen *et al.*, 2000).

In general, results from prospective studies are not as convincing as those from the less rigorous case-control or cross-sectional studies (Christen *et al.*, 2000). Overall, they demonstrate a compelling, although not yet conclusive argument to implicate elevated plasma homocysteine as a risk factor for CVD, independent of other known risk factors. One meta-analysis of 27 studies concluded that a raised homocysteine level (above the 90th–95th percentile) is associated with increased risk of fatal and non-fatal atherosclerotic vascular disease in the coronary (OR 1.7 [95%CI 1.5–1.9]), cerebral (2.5 [2.0–3.0]) and peripheral (6.8 [2.9–15.8]) circulations (Boushey *et al.*, 1995). This study also calculated, assuming a graded response, that a 5 μmol/L increment in plasma homocysteine would elevate risk of coronary artery disease by about one-third, similar to that imposed by an increase of 0.5 mmol/L in plasma cholesterol (Boushey *et al.*, 1995).

There is speculation as to the pathogenic process that might bring about such risk and it is fair to say that several mechanisms could account for the observed association. Homocysteine may directly cause CVD via a toxic effect on membranes or other cell structures or molecules. It might indirectly cause CVD by promoting the accumulation of SAH, which is a potent inhibitor of methylation reactions (Weir & Scott, 1998). It could function as a marker for some other folate, B_{12} or B_6 related event. Finally, it could be raised as a consequence rather than a cause of the atherogenic process (Christen *et al.*, 2000). Clearly, proof of a causal effect between elevated plasma homocysteine and CVD is urgently needed. However, this requires demonstrating, in large multi-centre trials, that a strategy to lower plasma homocysteine will reduce the frequency of cardiovascular events.

Vitamin supplementation to lower plasma homocysteine

Many studies now show that many apparently healthy normal individuals have plasma homocysteine levels that can be lowered by taking extra folic acid. The level of supplementation does not have to be high to achieve a decrease. A recent meta-analysis of these intervention trials (Homocysteine Lowering Trialists' Collaboration, 1998) indicated that supplementation with between 0.5 and 5.0 mg/day of folic acid over an average of 6 weeks caused a reduction of plasma homocysteine by between 25% and 35% (an approximate drop from 12 to 9 μmol/L). Addition of vitamin B_{12} to the regimen contributed a further 7% reduction while vitamin B_6

had no additional effect. This meta-analysis also concluded that, in general, folic acid supplements caused greater reduction in plasma homocysteine the higher the starting homocysteine level or the lower the starting plasma folate.

At present at least nine large randomised trials are underway in several countries (USA, UK, Norway, Canada and Australia) to test the efficacy of vitamin supplementation in the prevention of CVD (Eikelboom *et al.*, 1999). These trials differ with respect to disease manifestation (vascular disease, unstable angina, stroke) treatment regimen (folic acid alone, folic acid plus B_{12} and/or B_6, dosage variations), or outcome measurements (death, recurrent disease) (Eikelboom *et al.*, 1999). It is likely that the trials will have to last a number of years to act as a reasonable test of effectiveness, particularly those being carried out in the USA and Canada, where folic acid fortification has already reduced the prevalence of low folate status and hyperhomocysteinemia in the general population (Bostom & Garber, 2000).

Even if vitamin supplementation turns out to be an effective way of reducing the prevalence of CVD, this therapy is unlikely to become a successful public health strategy to prevent CVD. The issue of how to increase the folate status of the general population has already come under intense debate regarding the prevention of neural tube defects. The strategy adopted by the USA for the prevention of neural tube defects – fortification of grain – has successfully increased the folate status and reduced the plasma homocysteine of US citizens (Jacques *et al.*, 1999). The alternative strategy – promotion of lifestyle changes to increase consumption of dietary folate – may be more desirable but would be far more difficult to set in place and the success of such a choice would ultimately depend on the ability of natural foods to deliver sufficient folate to achieve the required status.

References

Bostom, A.G. & Garber, C. (2000) Endpoints for homocysteine-lowering trials. *Lancet*, **355**, 511–12.

Boushey, C.J., Beresford, S.A., Omenn, G.S. & Motulsky, A.G. (1995) A quantitative assessment of plasma homocysteine as a risk factor for vascular disease. *JAMA*, **274**, 1049–57.

Christen, W.G., Ajani, U.A., Glynn, R.J., Hennekens, C.H. (2000) Blood levels of homocysteine and increased risks of cardiovascular disease. *Arch. Intern. Med.*, **160**, 422–34.

Eikelboom, J.W., Lonn, E., Genest, J., Hankey, G. & Yusuf, S. (1999) Homocyst(e)ine and cardiovascular disease: A critical review of the epidemiological evidence. *Ann. Intern. Med.*, **131**, 363–75.

Finkelstein, J.D. (2000) Homocysteine: A history in progress. *Nutr. Rev.*, **58**, 193–204.

Frosst, P., Blom, H.J., Milos, R., Goyette, P., Sheppard, C.A., Matthews, R.G., Boers, G.J.H., den Heijer, M., Kluijmans, L.A., van den Heuvel, L.P. & Rozen, R. (1995) A candidate genetic risk factor for vascular disease: A common mutation in methylene-tetrahydrofolate reductase. *Nature Genet.*, **10**, 111–13.

Homocysteine Lowering Trialists' Collaboration (1998) Lowering blood homocysteine with folic acid based supplements: Meta-analysis of randomized trials. *BMJ*, **316**, 894–8.

Jacques, P.F., Selhub, J., Bostom, A.G., Wilson, P.W. & Rosenberg, I.H. (1999) The effect of folic acid fortification on plasma folate and total homocysteine concentrations. *New Eng. J. Med.*, **340**, 1449–54.

McCully, K.S. (1969) Vascular pathology of homocysteinemia: Implications for the pathogenesis of arteriosclerosis. *Am. J. Pathol.*, **56**, 111–28.

McKeever, M.P., Weir, D.G., Molloy, A., Scott, J.M. (1991) Betaine-homocysteine methyltransferase: Organ distribution in man, pig and rat and subcellular distribution in the rat. *Clin Sci.*, **81**, 551–6.

Mudd, S.H., Finklestein, J.D., Irreverre, F. & Laster, L. (1964) Homocystinuria: an enzymatic defect. *Science*, **143**, 1443–5.

Mudd, S.H., Skovby, F., Levy, H.L., Pettigrew, K.D., Wilken, B., Pyeritz, R.E., Andria, G., Boers, G.H., Bromberg, I.L. & Cerone, R. (1985) The natural history of homocystinuria due to cystathionine-beta-synthase deficiency. *Am. J. Hum. Genet.*, **37**, 1–31.

Refsum, H., Helland, S. & Ueland, P.M. (1985) Radioenzymic determination of homocysteine in plasma and urine. *Clin. Chem.*, **31**, 624–8.

Selhub, J., Jacques, P.F., Bostom, A.G., D'Agostino, R.B., Wilson, P.W.F., Belanger, A.J., O'Leary, D.H., Wolf, P.A., Schaefer, E.J. & Rosenberg, I.H. (1993) Vitamin status and intake as primary determinants of homocysteinemia in an elderly population. *JAMA.*, **270**, 2693–8.

Ueland, P.M., Refsum, H., Stabler, S.P., Malinow, M.R., Anderson, A., Allen, R.H. (1993) Total homocysteine in plasma or serum: Methods and clinical applications. *Clin Chem.*, **39**, 1764–79.

Ueland, P.M. & Refsum, H. (1989) Plasma homocysteine, a risk factor for vascular disease: Plasma levels in health, disease and drug therapy. *J. Lab. Clin. Med.*, **114**, 473–501.

Weir, D.G. & Scott, J.M. (1998) Homocysteine as a risk factor for cardiovascular and related disease: Nutritional implications. *Nutr. Res. Rev.*, **11**, 311–38.

7

DIETARY STRATEGIES TO PREVENT AND TREAT OBESITY

SUSAN A. JEBB

Introduction

Obesity is one of the greatest public health problems of the modern world. It is an independent risk factor for premature death and is strongly associated with a range of other conditions which are themselves risk factors for chronic disease, notably hyperlipidaemia, hypertension and insulin resistance.

Dietary strategies are a critical element in both the prevention and treatment of obesity and must be geared towards the achievement of a healthy weight and a reduction in the risk of co-morbid conditions. This chapter will consider the use of low fat diets to aid weight control and the debate over substitution of dietary fat, especially saturated fat, with carbohydrate, mono-unsaturated fats or protein to improve the metabolic profile.

In recent years obesity (defined as a body mass index greater than 30 kg/m^2) has emerged as a worldwide epidemic, affecting an estimated 7% of the adult population (Seidell, 1999). In developing countries obesity often co-exists with under-nutrition, and in developed and developing countries alike obesity is associated with a substantial burden of ill-health (WHO, 1998). Large prospective studies in the USA show that obesity is linked to a more than two-fold increased risk of premature death (Calle *et al.*, 1999). Obesity is an independent risk factor for disease, but it is also strongly associated with components of the metabolic syndrome, especially hyperlipidaemia, hypertension and insulin resistance. Obese people suffer increased morbidity from mechanical disorders including osteoarthritis, back pain and respiratory problems such as breathlessness and sleep apnoea (Jung, 1997). There is also a link to impaired mental health. This association is probably not causal, but instead reflects the discrimination suffered by obese people in cultures where leanness is highly regarded. Together this places a growing burden on health care systems and budgets and on business due to time off work, sick pay and early retirement, and results in personal, economic and social penalties to the obese individuals and their families.

Low fat diets and weight control

Obesity only develops when energy intake exceeds energy expenditure over a prolonged period. Intake and expenditure are governed both by genetic factors and by individual behaviours, which may themselves be influenced by environmental circumstances. The recent upsurge in the prevalence of obesity suggests that environmental factors are unmasking a latent genetic susceptibility to obesity – a classic gene-environment interaction (Jebb, 1999).

Over the last 50 years or so there has been a marked increase in the proportion of fat in the diet (MAFF, 1991) and this is associated with a reduced ability to match energy intake to energy needs (Prentice & Jebb, 1995). Experimental studies in animals and man have shown that when exposed to a high fat, energy dense diet, individuals readily over-eat, a phenomenon described as passive over-consumption (Prentice & Poppitt, 1996). In contrast reductions in dietary fat are associated with modest spontaneous weight loss. A recent meta-analysis of studies ranging from 3 to 12 months' duration showed a weighted mean weight loss relative to the control group of 2.55 kg (95% confidence interval – 1.5 to 3.5 kg. P<0.0001) (Astrup *et al.*, 2000). These *ad libitum* diets provide an effective strategy for the prevention of weight gain, but sustained and clinically significant weight loss usually requires additional strategies to limit total energy intake. This may include reductions in portion size, eating frequency or adjunctive drug therapy.

In overweight or obese individuals weight losses in excess of 5–10% of initial body weight are associated with clinically significant reductions in a number of metabolic risk factors (Table 7.1) (SIGN, 1996). However, since the aim of obesity management is to improve health, there may be scope to maximise these benefits by careful attention to the precise nature of the diet, especially the proportion of macronutrients.

Table 7.1 Benefits of 10 kg weight loss in 100 kg subject.

Mortality	20–25% decrease in premature mortality
Blood pressure	10 mmHg decrease in systolic pressure 20 mmHg decrease in diastolic pressure
Lipids	10% decrease in total cholesterol 15% decrease in LDL-cholesterol 8% increase in HDL-cholesterol 30% decrease in triglycerides
Diabetes	Reduces risk of developing NIDDM by 50% 30–50% decrease in elevated blood glucose 15% decrease in HbA1c

Impact of diet selection on obesity-related disease

The principal macronutrients in the diet are fat and carbohydrate and, at a population level, there is a clear reciprocity between them (Bolton-Smith & Woodward, 1994). In most experimental low fat interventions there has been a compensatory increase in the proportion of carbohydrate in the diet. Under iso-energetic conditions, this shift in the macronutrient composition of the diet is associated with an increase in triglycerides and a decrease in HDL-cholesterol, which implies a deterioration in the metabolic profile. However, the clinical significance of these changes is unclear. Indeed it has been argued that these effects are a transient consequence of acute changes in diet composition and are offset by the weight loss which accompanies a reduction in the proportion of dietary fat. This is supported by data from a study of patients with hyperlipaemia in which the dietary fat content was decreased from 35 to 15% energy (Schaefer *et al.*, 1995). Initially body weight was maintained and after 6 weeks total cholesterol was reduced by 13% and LDL-cholesterol by 17%, but HDL-cholesterol decreased by 23% and plasma triglyceride increased by 47%. Subsequently the subjects consumed an *ad libitum* diet of similar composition for 10–12 weeks. During this period weight decreased by 3.6 kg and this was associated with further reductions in LDL-cholesterol and a normalisation of plasma triglycerides and the ratio of HDL-cholesterol to total cholesterol.

In an attempt to offset the detrimental short-term metabolic effects of high carbohydrate diets a recent study has tested the substitution of fat with protein (Skov *et al.*, 1999). Subjects were recommended to reduce the proportion of fat in their diet to 30% by energy and in one group the proportion of carbohydrate was increased (58% by energy) with protein held constant (12% by energy) and in the second the proportion of protein (25% by energy) was increased with carbohydrate constant (45% by energy). Mean weight loss after six months was significantly greater in the high protein group relative to the high carbohydrate group (8.9 versus 5.1 kg, p <0.001), perhaps as a consequence of the greater satiating properties of protein relative to fat or carbohydrate (Rolls *et al.*, 1988). After three months plasma triglycerides had decreased in the high protein group by 0.37 mmol/l (p = 0.001) but increased in the high carbohydrate group by approximately 0.16 mmol/l. At six months the trend in triglycerides was similar but the difference between groups was not significant. Total and HDL-cholesterol decreased in both groups at each time-point, but there were no significant differences between the two groups.

These changes in the metabolic profile reflect the combined impact of weight loss and changes in the macronutrient content of the diet. This data suggests that substitution of fat with protein, primarily from lean meat and low fat dairy products, may be a useful strategy for the treatment of obesity, particularly since it allows greater dietary variety than conventional low fat/high carbohydrate diets. However, the longer-term health effects of such high protein intakes need further investigation.

In spite of the current preponderance of low fat diets there are a number of proponents of dietary strategies which focus exclusively on the substitution of saturated fat with mono-unsaturated fats (Katan *et al.*, 1997). The rationale for this approach stems from dietary intervention programmes to reduce cardiovascular risk and it is clear that there are metabolic benefits with respect to plasma lipids. For example, a meta-analysis has shown that under experimental conditions the iso-energetic substitution of saturated with mono-unsaturated fats in patients with type 2 diabetes is associated with a mean reduction of 0.36 mmol/l (19%) in triglycerides and an increase in HDL-cholesterol of 0.05 mmol/l (4%) relative to low fat/high carbohydrate diets (Garg, 1998). However, in public health terms, advocating low saturated/high mono-unsaturated fatty acid diets, with no overall reduction in the proportion of fat, is unlikely to offset the passive over-consumption associated with high fat diets. Long term prospective studies are required to evaluate the metabolic benefits of modest weight loss on a low fat diet relative to the improved lipid profile on a high mono-unsaturated fat diet.

In comparison with fat, studies of the health impact of different carbohydrate sources have received less attention in the context of weight loss. A recent European multi-centre intervention study compared weight loss and metabolic fitness in three groups of subjects (Saris *et al.*, 2000). The control group maintained their fat intake (36% by energy) and two further groups decreased the proportion of fat in their diet (approximately 27% by energy) and increased the proportion of carbohydrate. The latter two groups differed in the relative contribution of simple sugars to the total carbohydrate intake. After six months, weight loss in the low fat/low sugar group was -0.9 ± 3.6 kg compared to -1.8 ± 3.2 kg in the low fat/high sugar group. Weight losses in the two groups were not significantly different and both groups lost significantly more weight than the control group. Given the very small absolute weight change it is perhaps not surprising that there were no significant changes in blood lipids or insulin between the groups. However, in the longer term, there is evidence that the type of carbohydrate may have important effects on health, independent of body weight. Several epidemiological studies have now shown a graded decrease in cardiovascular disease risk with increased intake of wholegrain and low glycaemic index foods (Liu *et al.*, 1999, 2000). Such diets are also associated with a reduced risk of developing type 2 diabetes (Salmeron *et al.*, 1997a, b). Together this would suggest that obese patients should be advised to incorporate wholegrain foods with a high fibre content and low glycaemic index into their eating plan.

Finally, there is good evidence that diets rich in fruit and vegetables are associated with a decreased risk of cardiovascular disease and this is usually attributed to their antioxidant properties. Although there are no randomised trials where increases in fruit and vegetable consumption have been employed as a sole strategy for weight management, it would be anticipated that increasing fruit and vegetable intake would decrease the energy density of the diet and thus enhance appetite control. Additionally, such diets may have independent benefits with respect to hypertension, reducing both systolic and diastolic blood pressure. For example, in the DASH trial, subjects randomised to a diet rich in fruits and vegetables (approximately 9 servings per day) showed significant decreases in blood pressure, independent of changes in weight or salt intake (Appel *et al.*, 1997). The effects were greatest in the group also randomised to a low fat diet (27% fat versus 37% in the control group) perhaps because of additional benefits associated with an increased calcium intake from low fat dairy products.

Conclusion

There is now good evidence that at public health level we can develop dietary strategies to prevent obesity, which reduce the risk of weight gain and concomitantly decrease the risk of the metabolic diseases associated with obesity. A prudent diet will limit total fat to 30% or less by energy, focusing especially on reductions in saturated fat, and will allow modest portions of protein (up to 25% by energy), plentiful carbohydrate, especially from wholegrain sources, and at least five servings per day of fruits and vegetables. The treatment of patients who are already obese will continue to require more intensive intervention, but even in this group the greatest challenge is not so much the initial phase of weight loss but the ongoing need to prevent weight regain.

References

Appel, L.J., Moore, T.J., Obarzanek, E. *et al.* (1997) A clinical trial of the effects of dietary patterns on blood pressure. *N. Eng. J. Med.*, **336**, 1117-24.

Astrup, A., Ryan, L., Grunwald, G., *et al.* (2000) The role of dietary fat in body fatness: evidence from a preliminary meta-analysis of ad libitum low fat dietary intervention studies. *Brit. J. Nutr.*, **83**, S25-S32.

Bolton-Smith, C. & Woodward, M. (1994) Dietary composition and fat to sugar ratios in relation to obesity. *Int. J. Obes.*, **18**, 820-28.

Calle, E.E., Thun, M.J., Petrelli, J.M., Rodriguez, C. & Heath, C.W. (1999) Body mass index and mortality in a prospective cohort of US adults. *N. Eng. J. Med.*, **341**, 1097-105.

Garg, A. (1998) High-monounsaturated-fat diets for patients with diabetes mellitus: a meta-analysis. *Am. J. Clin. Nutr.*, **67**, 577S-82S.

Jebb. S.A. (1999) Obesity: from molecules to man. *Proc. Nutr. Soc.*, **58**, 1-14.

Jung, R. (1997) Obesity as a disease. *Br. Med. Bull.*, **53**, 307-21.

Katan, M., Grundy, S. & Willett, W. (1997) Beyond low-fat diets. *N. Eng. J. Med.*, **337**, 563-6.

Liu, S., Stampfer, M.J., Hu, F.B. *et al.* (1999) Whole-grain consumption and risk of coronary heart disease: results from the Nurses' Health Study. *Am. J. Clin. Nutr.*, **70**, 412-19.

Liu, S., Willett, W.C., Stampfer, M.J. *et al* (2000) A prospective study of dietary glycemic load, carbohydrate intake and risk of coronary heart disease in US women. *Am. J. Clin. Nutr.*, **71**, 1455-61.

MAFF (1991) *Fifty years of the National Food Survey*. The Stationery Office, London.

Prentice, A.M. & Jebb, S.A. (1995) Obesity in Britain: Gluttony or Sloth? *BMJ*, **311**, 437-9.

Prentice, A.M. & Poppitt, S.D. (1996) Importance of energy density and macronutrients in the regulation of energy intake. *Int. J. Obes.*, **20**, S18-S23.

Rolls, B.J., Hetherington, M. & Burley, V.J. (1988) The specificity of satiety: the influence of different macronutrient contents on the development of satiety. *Physiology and Behaviour*, **43**, 145-53.

Salmeron, J., Manson, J.E., Stampfer, M.J., Colditz, G.A., Wing, A.L. & Willett, W.C. (1997a) Dietary fiber, glycemic load, and risk of non-insulin dependent diabetes mellitus in women. *J. Am. Med. Assoc.*, **277**, 472-7.

Salmeron, J., Ascherio, A., Rimm, E.B. *et al.* (1997b) Dietary fiber, glycemic load, and risk of NIDDM in men. *Diabetes Care*, **20**, 545-50.

Saris, W.H.M., Astrup, A., Prentice, A.M. *et al.* (2000) Randomised controlled trial of changes in dietary carbohydrate/fat ratio and simple vs. complex carbohydrates on body weight and blood lipids: the CARMEN study. *Int. J. Obes.*, **24**, 1310–18.

Schaefer, E.J., Lichtenstein, A.H., Lamon-Fava, S. *et al.* (1995) Body weight and low density lipoprotein cholesterol changes after consumption of a low-fat ad libitum diet. *J. Am. Med. Assoc.*, **274**, 1450–55.

Seidell J.C. (1999) Obesity: a growing problem. *Acta. Pediatr. Scanda.*, **428S**, 46–50.

SIGN (1996) Obesity in Scotland. Integrating prevention with weight management. *Royal College of Physicians*, Edinburgh.

Skov, A.R., Toubro, S., Ronn, B., Holm, L. & Astrup, A. (1999) Randomised trial on protein vs carbohydrate in ad libitum fat reduced diet for the treatment of obesity. *Int. J. Obes.*, **23**, 528–36.

WHO (1998) *Obesity. Preventing and Managing the Global Epidemic.* World Health Organisation, Geneva.

8

PHYSICAL ACTIVITY, EXERCISE AND WEIGHT CONTROL: MOVEMENT FOR MANAGEMENT?

KENNETH R. FOX

Overweight and obesity are growing at an alarming rate and their association with increased risk of coronary heart disease, diabetes, colon cancer, joint and respiratory disorders, and reduced physical fitness currently make them probably the most serious threat to public health. When overweight and obesity are considered, for most people including the lay public and health professionals, food intake comes to mind. There is a strong belief that obesity results from overeating or a malfunction in metabolic control. Lack of activity is rarely attributed as a major causal role and a common view is that exercise has a negligible effect on energy balance. The view that the 300 kcals in a chocolate bar take only 30 seconds to consume but 30 minutes to exercise away provides a powerful disincentive.

In the past decade, research evidence has accumulated to establish the critical role that exercise and physical activity play in both health and long-term weight management and this is slowly filtering through to health professionals, commercial slimming organisations and the general public. This chapter provides a brief synopsis of the nature and strength of this evidence and its implications for exercise recommendations. Issues are also raised for future consideration of research and practice. Throughout the chapter the terms 'physical activity' and 'exercise' are used. Physical activity has the broader meaning of the two and encapsulates all significant bodily movement engaged in through the daily routine such as housework, walking and cycling as a form of transport, shopping and active hobbies. Exercise is confined to those physical activities (which might include some from this list) that are undertaken with the intention of improving aspects of health, fitness or weight management. Exercise is the main focus of almost all of the summarised research discussed in this chapter, but lifestyle activity may also have an important role.

Exercise and health

Often the effectiveness of exercise is judged solely on its contribution to weight loss. However, its greatest contribution is in the reduction in risk of early disease and death. Active living represents the normal state and it is hardly surprising that sedentary habits lead to reduced physical function and increased risk of several health problems. Sedentary living doubles the risk of all-cause mortality (Powell *et al.*, 1987; Berlin & Colditz, 1990), and this is similar to the risks carried by smoking, hypertension, and dislipidemia. Health organisations world-wide now regard physical inactivity as an independent risk factor for coronary heart disease and stroke (Killoran *et al.*, 1994; US Department of Health and Human Services, 1996; World Health Organisation, 1995). Physical activity has other benefits including the management of diabetes, reduction in risk of some cancers, improved physical fitness and psychological well-being (Biddle *et al.*, 2000).

Overweight and obese people tend to fall in the least active sector of the population and are also at heightened risk of problems such as cardiorespiratory disease and diabetes, against which physical activity has a protective effect. This is particularly the case for middle-aged men with abdominal obesity and susceptibility to metabolic syndrome. Recent research (Lee *et al.*, 1999) suggests that it is possible to be fit and healthy even when overweight or mildly obese, so long as it is accompanied by regular exercise.

Although the main improvement in mortality rate seen with exercise appears to be due to reduction in cardiovascular disease, there is also some evidence that increased activity reduces incidence of colon cancers and breast and endometrial cancers in obese women (Rissanen & Fogelholm, 1999). There is also promising evidence that exercise can have a positive impact on mental well-being and may be a useful medium for the treatment of depression (Mutrie, 2000) and low self-esteem (Fox, 2000), problems which are heightened in obese women. The accumulated evidence of the benefits of exercise for the health of overweight and obese people clearly indicates that it has to be considered as a critical element of any prevention or treatment programme regardless of its effect on weight loss.

Exercise and weight loss

There have been many reviews of studies investigating the effect of exercise on weight loss. Many of the early papers have not fully described the exercise programme or have adopted a prescription model that is now outdated, and so it is difficult to fully evaluate the effectiveness of best practice for body composition change or weight loss. However, there is a general consensus among reviewers that is expressed in the most recent review conducted by Wing (1999). Exercise by itself results in modest weight loss in the order of 0.5 kg to 1 kg per month. This is a small amount in comparison to reduced calorie diets and is often disappointing to the patient. However, exercise is effective over extended periods. For example, a daily walking programme creates the energy deficit of the equivalent of about 5–6 kg per year. Greatest weight loss is seen in programmes that involve both dietary restriction and an exercise protocol. Weight loss due to exercise seems to be less in females than males, possibly because there is a stronger effect on abdominal versus femoral fat deposition.

Reviews indicate that there this is greater loss of fat and conservation of lean tissue (mainly muscle mass) when exercise is added to a dietary routine. This becomes important to resting metabolic rate which is largely determined by the amount of muscle tissue and which for normal activity levels creates around 60% of daily energy expenditure. A greater muscle bulk will produce greater energy expenditure even when the body is at rest. Recently, this has initiated greater interest in the use of resistance exercise to increase muscle mass and also maximise maintenance of muscle mass during dieting. One study using magnetic resonance imaging indicated no loss of muscle tissue during weight loss in obese women undergoing a resistance exercise programme and diet (Ross *et al.*, 1995).

Although exercise is unable to compete with hypocaloric diets for weight loss, it should be considered an essential part of any programme as it increases weight loss, preserves muscle tissue and provides opportunity to habituate the individual to healthier lifestyle patterns that have a better prognosis for long-term weight management and health.

Exercise and sustained weight loss

The greatest challenge is the maintenance of weight loss. Long-term success is only achieved by a small percentage of those who attempt to keep their weight down. King and Tribble (1991) estimated the effects of programmes that incorporated follow-up measures of at least 6 months. The average sustained weight loss was 4.0 kg in four diet-only programmes, 4.9 kg in five exercise-only programmes, and 7.2 kg in three diet and exercise programmes. In the more recent review of Wing (1999) the results of six randomised control weight loss trials that had incorporated an exercise programme were summarised. Three of the studies showed significantly greater long-term weight loss when compared to the diet only groups.

Further research is needed to substantiate this effect. There are probably several mechanisms involved in addition to the extra energy expended. For example, exercise may help the maintenance of a higher muscle mass and metabolic rate. Additionally, exercise success and the accompanying improvements in self-perceptions may empower individuals to improve eating habits and reduce energy intake.

Exercise and prevention of weight gain

The potential role of physical activity as a causal agent in obesity development was graphically brought to light by Prentice and Jebb (1995). Using national survey data they plotted indirect indicators of inactivity such as time spent watching television and number of cars per household against the rapid rise in obesity seen in the past 20 years. A strong positive relationship emerged that was not observed with dietary and fat intake data. This is supported by a recent study involving several European countries that established a positive graded relationship between time spent watching television and body mass index group (Martinez-Gonzalez *et al.*, 1999). Cross-sectional data sets have also consistently shown an association between degree of overweight and physical activity (Centres of Disease Control, 1995; Prescott-Clarke & Primatesta , 1997).

There is a wealth of incidental evidence indicating that increased wealth and advances in technology have led to small but critical secular reductions in average daily energy expenditure. The widespread availability of labour-saving devices at home and at work, fewer active occupations, availability of motorised transport and the attractiveness of wall-to-wall electronic home entertainment have taken away much of the incidental activity in our daily routines. It is not far fetched to see that this would contribute to weight increase, particularly in those with genetic predispositions for obesity.

There is some evidence to show that those who counteract this secular tendency towards energy saving by engaging in compensatory recreational exercise can at least attenuate if not prevent the weight gain that is typical with increasing age. Those who report physical activity such as golf, jogging, cycling and walking through middle age exhibit less weight gain than their non-active counterparts (Williamson *et al.*, 1993). More rigorous data are provided by seven prospective studies that have investigated the relationship between physical activity over at least five year periods and subsequent weight change. The general consensus from these studies (Di Pietro, 1999) is that maintenance of an exercise programme throughout middle age substantially reduces the amount of weight that is typically gained. In some groups this can be as much as 3–7 times reduced risk of substantial weight gain in women.

There seems to be good evidence from several sources that points towards reduced activity and daily energy expenditure as a contributing factor to the dramatic growth in obesity. Furthermore, those who counteract this trend by participation in activities such as recreational sport, exercise sessions, walking or cycling appear to be more successful at preventing the gain in weight that is typical of middle age. Of course, they also experience many health benefits at the same time. From a public health perspective, exercise cannot be ignored as a primary vehicle for the prevention of obesity and other diseases.

Physical activity recommendations

The US Surgeon General and the Department of Health have issued similar recommendations for physical activity for health. This followed extensive reviews of existing research evidence. Every adult, regardless of whether or not they are overweight, should aim to accumulate 30 minutes of moderate intensity physical activity equivalent to brisk walking on at least 5 days per week. Moderate intensity exercise is sufficiently exertive to increase body temperature, produce a mild sweat, but still remains comfortable and allows conversation. Such a programme would induce improvements in physical fitness and metabolic health in those who have done little previous activity. In the case of obese people, this recommendation should be regarded as the long-term target after several months of build up that involves shorter walks of 10–15 minute periods at a comfortable pace and avoiding hills. The important factor in the early stages is to build up an activity routine.

In addition to a purposeful and planned exercise programme, it would be beneficial for those seeking weight loss or weight management to increase their levels of general movement throughout the day. More walking, less television watching and taking up active hobbies such as gardening may seem alien to modern culture but will significantly increase long-term energy expenditure. Energy expenditure is greatest when body weight is being moved, particularly against gravity as in stairs and slopes.

Obese individuals are among the least likely to voluntarily develop an exercise routine. This is hardly surprising given that many will have had exercise experiences in the past that have not been encouraging. Health professionals will be required to give substantial and sensitive support that will involve educating patients about the amount and type of activity required, how to build confidence in exercise settings, and how to develop exercise routines through a range of cognitive-behavioural strategies.

References

Berlin, J.A. & Colditz, G.A. (1990) A meta analysis of physical activity in the prevention of coronary heart disease. *Am. J. Epidemiol.*, **132**, 612–28.

Biddle, S.J.H., Fox K.R, & Boutcher, S.H. (eds) (2000) Physical activity and psychological well-being. Routledge, London.

Centres of Disease Control (1995) *Assessing Health Risks in America. The Behavioral Risk Factor Surveillance System (BRFSS) at a Glance*. Centres for Disease Control and Prevention, Atlanta, GA.

Di Pietro, L. (1999) Physical activity in the prevention of obesity: current evidence and research issues. *Med. Sci. Sport Ex.*, **31**, S542–6.

Fox, K.R. (2000) The influence of exercise on self-perceptions and self-esteem. In *Physical Activity and Psychological Well-being* (eds S.J.H. Biddle, K.R. Fox, & S.H. Boutcher), pp. 88–117. Routledge, London.

Killoran, A.J. Fentem, P., & Casperson C. (eds) (1994) *Moving on: International Perspectives on Promoting Physical Activity*. Health Education Authority, London.

King, A.C. & Tribble, D.L. (1991) The role of exercise in weight regulation in nonathletes. *Sports Med.*, **11**, 331–49.

Lee, C.D., Blair, S.N. & Jackson, A.S. (1999) Cardiorespiratory fitness, body composition, and all-cause mortality in men. *Am. J. Clin. Nutr.*, **69**, 373–80.

Martinez-Gonzalez, M.A., Martinez, J.A., Hu, F.B., Gibney, M.J. & Kearney, J. (1999) Physical inactivity, sedentary lifestyle and obesity in the European Union. *Int. J. Obes.*, **23**, 1192–201.

Mutrie, N. (2000) The relationship between physical activity and clinically defined depression. In: *Physical Activity and Psychological Well-being* (eds S.J.H. Biddle, K.R. Fox, & S.H. Boutcher), pp. 446-62. Routledge, London.

Powell, K.E., Thompson, P.D., Casperson, C.J. & Kendrick, J.S. (1987) Physical activity and the incidence of coronary heart disease. *Ann. Rev. Pub. Health*, **8**, 253-87.

Prentice, A.M. & Jebb, S. (1995) Obesity in Britain: Gluttony or sloth. *BMJ*, **311**, 437-9.

Prescott-Clarke, P. & Primatesta, P. (1997) *Health Survey for England, 1995: Findings (Vol. 1)*. The Stationery Office, London.

Rissanen, A. & Fogelholm, M. (1999) Physical activity in the prevention and treatment of other morbid conditions and impairments associated with obesity: current evidence and research issues. *Med. Sci. Sport Ex.*, **31**, S635-45.

Ross, R. Pedwell, H. & Rissanen, J. (1995) Response of total and regional lean tissue and skeletal muscle to a program of energy restriction and resistance exercise. *Int. J. Obes.*, **19**, 781-7.

US Department of Health and Human Services (PHS) (1996) Physical activity and health: A report of the Surgeon General (Executive Summary). Pittsburgh, PA.

WHO (1995) Exercise for health. WHO/FMS Committee on Physical Activity for Health. *Bulletin of the World Health Organisation*, **73**, 135-6.

Williamson, D.F., Madans, J., Anda, R.F. *et al.* (1993) Recreational physical activity and ten-year weight change in a US national cohort. *Int. J. Obes.*, **17**, 279-86.

Wing, R.R. (1999) Physical activity in the treatment of the adulthood overweight and obesity: current evidence and research issues. *Med. Sci. Sport Ex.*, **31**, S547-52.

9

COGNITIVE-BEHAVIOURAL INTERVENTIONS FOR OBESITY

CAROLYN EDWARDS

Introduction

The original application of behavioural treatments to weight management stemmed from the belief that abnormal eating and activity behaviours were the cause of obesity. Based on the principles of learning theory, it was hypothesised that the application of behavioural techniques would reverse dysfunctional eating and activity habits allowing weight to return to a 'normal' level (Ferster *et al.*, 1962). Although it is now widely assumed that excessive eating and insufficient exercise are but two components of a complex biopsychosocial model of obesity, behavioural approaches (and latterly cognitive-behavioural approaches) continue to be viewed as important components of modern day weight management programmes. Aside from surgical treatments, cognitive-behaviour therapy (CBT) together with advice on nutrition and exercise offers the most consistently effective results in the treatment of obesity.

Brief history of psychological approaches

Health professionals have become increasingly aware that the mere pro-vision of advice on healthy eating and activity does not necessarily result in behaviour change (Glanz, 1985). Clinical and health psychologists' contribution to the obesity field has been the application of psychological theory and principles focusing on *how* individuals can be helped to make behavioural changes. Starting with Stuart in 1967, initial results of behavioural interventions were impressive. Largely ignoring nutritional aspects, and focusing instead on changing eating patterns (e.g. where and when foods are eaten), early studies indicated that behaviour modification was more effective than nutritional education (McReynolds *et al.*, 1976).

Behavioural treatments

The behavioural approach grew out of learning theory. As applied to obesity, it was based on the following assumptions:

(1) Eating and exercise behaviours affect body weight

Originally obesity was thought to be caused by abnormal eating and exercise behaviours. Although we have moved on to a multifactorial view of obesity and these behaviours are no longer thought to be especially abnormal, energy balance still holds the key to weight change. While the behavioural approach does not rule out genetic, metabolic or hormonal influences and recognises the impact of the individual's past history (e.g. culture/family influences), behaviour therapy is directed towards the modification of *current* eating and exercise behaviours in order to achieve a negative energy balance.

(2) Eating and exercise behaviours are learned behaviours

Applying the principles of classical and operant conditioning, it is posited that behaviours are learned through their repeated association with certain antecedent or simultaneous events (classical conditioning) and, if followed by a positive consequence are likely to occur again (operant conditioning). Thus, a dysfunctional eating habit (behaviour) is triggered by aspects of the situation with which it has become associated (e.g. the sight or smell of food) and/or strengthened by the consequences of performing the behaviour (e.g. alleviation of discomfort).

(3) Behaviours can be modified by changing the environment or changing the individual's response to his/her environment

Behavioural interventions aim to weaken such associations by manipulating the stimuli which trigger the behaviour or by modifying the individual's reaction to them. These will be described in detail later.

Cognitive-behavioural approaches

During the late 1960s and early 1970s, the importance of individual differences and cognitive factors became increasingly evident. Meichenbaum (1975) suggested that behaviour change could be brought about by changing the instructions patients gave themselves, away from negative and maladaptive thoughts to more positive self-talk. The field of behaviour therapy, which had focused strictly on the observable, began to take the role of cognitive processes into account. Cognitive-behaviour therapy emphasised the importance of internal (cognitive) processes and focused on the link between thoughts, feelings and behaviours.

While cognitive theory views thoughts and beliefs as integral to the development and maintenance of psychiatric disorders (notably depression and anxiety), obesity treatments have tended to selectively incorporate some of the techniques, namely identifying and modifying self-defeating cognitions. As a consequence, so-called cognitive-behavioural interventions for the treatment of obesity bear little resemblance to the well-defined treatment approaches for other disorders. Cognitive-behaviour therapy as it is applied to weight management is a method for systematically modifying eating, exercise and other behaviours thought to contribute to or maintain obesity (Stunkard, 1996).

What is the evidence that psychological interventions are effective for the treatment of obesity?

In a review of randomised clinical trials of behavioural treatments for obesity over the past three decades, Wadden and Foster (2000) have shown that total weight losses have more than doubled since behavioural interventions were first applied. Since average weight losses per week have remained relatively constant over the past 20 years, at about 0.5 kg (1 lb) a week, Wadden and Foster have attributed the greater total weight losses in more recent studies to longer treatment interventions, rather than the additional contribution of cognitive components. In 1974, average behavioural interventions were 8 weeks compared to an average of 22 weeks in studies between 1991 and 1995.

In the review, current cognitive-behavioural interventions are shown to produce weight losses of approximately 9% of initial weight in 20 weeks of treatment, reducing to around 6% at one year follow-up. These indicate favourable results when judged by the new criteria for success proposed by the Institute of Medicine (1995), which recommends a minimum 5% reduction in initial weight, maintained for at least a year.

Cognitive-behavioural approaches for obesity

CBT approaches have traditionally been conducted in a group setting (10–20 participants), with treatment individualised through lessons on problem solving where the individual is able to focus on his/her specific problem areas. Group interventions may be conducted by one therapist (usually a clinical psychologist) or a team of therapists (e.g. clinical psychologist, exercise physiologist and dietitian).

Most of the various approaches termed 'cognitive-behavioural' include several core components, briefly detailed below. These include assessment, goal setting, self-monitoring, functional analysis, stimulus control, problem solving, cognitive restructuring and relapse prevention. While early behavioural interventions did not include nutritional advice, dietary education is usually included as a component of modern day CBT programmes. Similarly, most CBT programmes also include an exercise component where increasing lifestyle and programmed activities and decreasing sedentary behaviours (e.g. watching television) are emphasised. Sometimes, although not always, programmes include interventions for body image, binge eating and stress management.

Assessment

Although most interventions for obesity offer a single approach for all patients, individual assessment is considered essential in understanding the factors contributing to and maintaining the individual's weight gain. Assessments of the individual's weight history, health, current psychological functioning, social context, goals and expectations of treatment are important to achieve a multifactorial formulation of the problem and in assessing readiness to change.

Goal setting

The health and psychological benefits achieved with relatively small amounts of weight loss (Goldstein, 1992) have led to recommendations that the goals of obesity treatments change to encourage the individual to aim for modest weight losses, which can be maintained. This is not new to behavioural approaches, where one of the foundations is the learning principle of successive approximation – breaking a task into small achievable goals. Successful accomplishment of a goal provides the individual with a sense of mastery on which to build further small changes. Setting specific behavioural goals and monitoring their outcome continues to be an integral part of CBT programmes for weight management.

Self-monitoring

Self-monitoring has been the cornerstone of behavioural programmes. Keeping a food and activity diary may serve as an intervention in itself, as increased awareness may lead to reduced food intake. Few people keep an accurate account of what and when they eat and a written record, if it can be done, provides a good basis for increasing awareness and planning for and monitoring change. Accurate self-monitoring helps to identify the actual amount of food consumed and when, and helps to identify the specific problem areas to be targeted in treatment.

Functional analysis

Functional analysis enables a detailed analysis of the occurrence of behaviours the individual wishes to change. Using the eating and activity diary, analysing the antecedents (cues) and the consequences (reinforcers) of a behaviour helps the individual to target aspects of his or her environment, or response to the environment, which can be modified. Eating can be triggered by one factor or a variety of factors in a chain of events.

Triggers or cues for eating can be external, e.g. the sight or smell of food, or internal, e.g. thoughts and feelings. Once identified, the individual may be taught methods of stimulus control, where he/she is taught to decrease exposure to the stimuli which trigger (inappropriate) eating, for example, not having high calorie snack foods available at home. In addition to decreasing the cues for undesirable eating and exercise behaviours, environmental changes can be made to *increase* the cues for *desirable* diet and exercise behaviours, e.g. buying more fruit and vegetables or putting training shoes next to the front door as a reminder to exercise.

In the longer term, it is more effective to eliminate the associations between stimuli and urges to eat, through exposing the individual to the trigger (e.g. looking at food) and inhibiting their usual response (i.e. eating). Exposure induces a dramatic increase in the urge to eat but this usually reduces over a 5–30 minute period, giving the person an experience of self-control. Exposure and response prevention has been shown to be a useful technique in reducing binge eating (Fairburn & Wilson, 1993).

Cognitive restructuring techniques

Cognitive restructuring describes the process of identifying, challenging and modifying unrealistic or maladaptive thoughts. Individuals are taught to record their automatic thoughts, find the evidence for and against these thoughts/beliefs and substitute more helpful alternatives. Unlike cognitive-behavioural interventions for psychiatric conditions, where working with the individual's thoughts and beliefs occurs throughout the treatment process, its application to weight management tends to focus on challenging unhelpful thoughts during the initial phase of setting weight loss goals (e.g. I'm only going to be happy if I'm a size 10) and when dealing with lapses (see below).

Relapse prevention

Preparing the individual to appreciate that lapses (slips) are a natural part of the change process, is an important component of cognitive-behavioural interventions. Individuals are taught to predict situations which might cause a lapse, and to problem solve thinking of coping strategies before high risk situations arise. When a lapse does occur, it is common for people in weight control programmes to fall into the 'black and white' thinking trap, where one slip is perceived as 'having blown it'. Individuals are taught to restructure a lapse as a learning experience and not as failure. Continuing self-monitoring and functional analysis helps to identify triggers which lead to the lapse and problem solve what might be done differently next time.

Managing body image, binge-eating and well-being

Cognitive-behavioural interventions have been used to improve body image satisfaction, reducing binge eating and/or improving well-being. Some researchers suggest taking the emphasis off weight loss completely and emphasising self-acceptance, improved body image, better nutrition and increased rates of physical activity (Wooley & Wooley, 1984; Garner & Wooley, 1991; Robison, 1997).

Typical cognitive–behavioural interventions in these 'new paradigm' obesity treatments include educational approaches to challenge the negative stereotypes regarding obesity, the identification and modification of negative thoughts and beliefs about physical appearance and exposure to avoided body image situations. In addition to improved body image satisfaction and self-esteem, an interesting artifact of studies using this approach has been improvements in self-reported eating habits despite not being addressed directly in treatment (Rosen *et al.*, 1995).

Interventions to improve body image may turn out to be a key component of treatments for overweight/obesity. Body image dissatisfaction correlates with both low mood and low self-esteem (Sarwer *et al.*, 1998) and may compromise compliance with treatment as it is strongly associated with behavioural avoidance (Cash, 1990).

While body image components are viewed as an important part of treatment for anorexia nervosa and bulimia nervosa, it is often thought to be more difficult to intervene with overweight subjects because of the implication of learning to accept oneself in spite of an appearance falling short of societal ideals. Interventions aimed at improving body image seem to be a fruitful area of research.

Limitations of CBT interventions for obesity

Although the use of CBT strategies has been helpful in improving short-term weight losses (up to one year), long-term success continues to be elusive. Factors which have been shown to improve the long-term maintenance of initial weight losses include longer interventions (Perri *et al.*, 1988), exercise (Colvin & Olson, 1984; Kayman *et al.*, 1990) and the continuation of self-monitoring (Wadden & Leitzia, 1992). The finding that weight is regained over time, although disappointing, is perhaps not surprising when compared to other chronic disorders such as diabetes or hypertension. Foster and Kendall (1994) recommend that the notion of a 'cure' be abandoned and that a chronic illness model with the emphasis on permanent lifestyle changes be adopted.

The future

There has been an increasing interest shown by non-psychologists in the adoption of psychological approaches (Rapoport, 1998). With the incidence of obesity ever increasing and the small numbers of clinical psychologists working in this field, new ways of disseminating skills are required. Training dietitians and other health professionals in the use of cognitive-behavioural approaches, developing self-help treatment manuals and combining pharmacological and cognitive-behavioural interventions are some of the most recent developments.

References

Cash, T.F. (1990) The psychology of physical appearance: aesthetics, attributes and images. In: *Body Images: Development, Deviance and Change* (eds T.F. Cash & T. Pruzinsky). Guilford Press, New York.

Colvin, R.H. & Olson, S.B. (1984) Winners revisited: An 18 month follow-up of our successful weight losers. *Addict. Behav.*, **9**, 305–6.

Fairburn, C.G. & Wilson, G.T. (1993) *Binge Eating: Nature, Assessment and Treatment*. Guilford Press, New York.

Ferster, C.B., Nurnberger, J.L. & Levitt, E.B. (1962) The control of eating. *J. Mathetics*, **1**, 87–109.

Foster, G.D. & Kendall, P.C. (1994) The realistic treatment of obesity: Changing the scales of success. *Clin. Psychol. Rev.*, **14**, 701–36.

Garner, D.M. & Wooley, S.C. (1991) Confronting the failure of behavioural and dietary treatments for obesity. *Clin. Psychol. Rev.*, **11**, 729–80.

Glanz, K. (1985) Nutrition education for risk factor reduction and patient education: A review. *Preventative Medicine*, **14**, 721–52.

Goldstein, D.J. (1992) Beneficial health effects of modest weight loss. *Int. J. Obes.*, **16**, 397–415.

Institute of Medicine (1995) *Weighing the options: Criteria for evaluating weight management programs*. Government Printing Office, Washington DC.

Kayman, S., Bruvold, W. & Stern, J.S. (1990) Maintenance and relapse after weight loss in women: Behavioural aspects. *Am. J. Clinical Nutr.*, **52**, 800–807.

Meichenbaum, D.H. (1975) Self-instructional methods. In: *Helping People Change: a Textbook of Methods* (eds F.H. Kanfer & A.P. Goldstein). Pergamon, New York.

McReynolds, W.T., Lutz, R.N., Paulsen, B.K. & Kohrs, M.B. (1976) Weight loss resulting from two behaviour modification procedures with nutritionists as therapists. *Behavior Therapy*, **7**, 283–91.

Perri, M., McAllister, D., Gange, J., Jordan, R.C., McAdoo, W.G. & Nezu, A.M. (1988) Effects of four maintenance programs on the long-term management of obesity. *J. Consult. Clin. Psychol.*, **56**, 529–34.

Rapoport, L. (1998) Integrating cognitive behavioural therapy into dietetic practice: a challenge for dietitians. *J. Human Nutr. Dietetics*, **9**, 227–47.

Robison, J. (1997) Weight management: shifting the paradigm. *J. Health Education*, **28**, 28–34.

Rosen, J.C, Orosan, P. & Reiter, J. (1995) Cognitive-behaviour therapy for negative body image in obese women. *Behavior Therapy*, **26**, 25–42.

Sarwer, D.B., Wadden, T.A. & Foster, G.D. (1998) Assessment of body image dissatisfaction in obese women: specificity, severity and clinical significance. *J. Consult. Clin. Psychol.*, **66**(4), 651–4.

Stuart, R. (1967) Behavioral control of overeating. *Behavior Therapy*, **5**, 357–65.

Stunkard, A.J. (1996) Current views on obesity. *Am. J. Med.*, **100**, 230–36.

Wadden, T.A. & Foster, G.D. (2000) Behavioural treatment of obesity. *Medical Clinics of North America*, **84**, 441–61.

Wadden, T.A. & Leitzia, K.A. (1992) Predictors of attrition and weight loss in persons treated by moderate and severe caloric restriction. In: *Treatment of the Seriously Obese Patient* (eds T.A. Wadden & T. Van Itallie). Guilford Press, New York.

Wooley, S.C. & Wooley, O.W. (1984) Should obesity be treated at all? In: *Eating and its Disorders* (eds A.J. Stunkard & E.J. Stellar). Raven, New York.

10

ASPECTS OF FETAL ORIGINS OF DISEASE

ALAN A. JACKSON

The traditional perception is that chronic diseases such as heart disease, diabetes and cancer arise because of a genetic predisposition which interacts with lifestyle factors operating during adult life. Thus, smoking, lack of exercise and an inappropriate diet increase the risk of the disease in those who are especially susceptible because of their genetic inheritance. However, it is now becoming increasingly clear that this orthodox position is not able to explain a large part of the variability in risk seen amongst individuals. Therefore there must be other important factors which play a powerful part. Studies in Southampton and elsewhere over the last fifteen years have identified one factor of substantial significance. This hypothesis has come to be known as the 'fetal origins of adult disease' enunciated by Barker (1998).

The hypothesis refines and extends observations which have been made earlier to show that an adverse early nutritional environment can permanently blight a fetus by modifying the development of its structure and function. These alterations which operate to enhance survival in the short term, lead to changes which increase the risk of disease later in life. Thus in epidemiological studies small size at birth or infancy is associated with increased risk of heart disease, diabetes, some cancers and mental ill-health. It was proposed and has now been shown, that metabolic behaviour is modified during growth in a way which later increases the sensitivity to other potential adverse influences in the environment. During early life nutrient exposure sets the capacity for the metabolic response in the fetus, thus when exposed to environmental stressors during adult life, the limited capacity to respond increases the risk of chronic disease (Jackson, 1996).

Effect of nutrient environment on the fetus

Population-based studies, human experimental studies and animal studies confirm that the nutrient environment which the mother provides for her developing fetus and nutritional exposure during early life have a profound impact on the susceptibility of an individual to the risk of chronic disease during adulthood. One important aspect of the hypothesis that is often overlooked is that the variation in risk is not simply a feature of the extremes of birth weight, the very light or the very heavy babies, but is graded across the entire birth weight distribution. Remarkably, within the normal range of birth weights (2.5 to 4.5 kg) there is a two to threefold difference in risk of developing heart disease or type 2 diabetes. There are graded differences in blood pressure, which can be found as early as 4 years of age and can persist and amplify throughout life. Similarly, using biochemical tests graded differences can be identified for insulin resistance and glucose tolerance, dyslipidaemia, with increased LDL and TAG and decreased HDL, and increased clotting (Barker, 1998). These intermediate markers are directly associated with increased mortality from cardiovascular disease, heart disease and stroke, and together with increased prevalence of central obesity, fully characterise a remarkable predisposition to syndrome X, with up to a tenfold difference in risk between the lightest and heaviest babies at birth. Although special tests can identify this difference in risk during early childhood, it becomes more obvious with age, interacting with other lifestyle factors to express itself as frank disease.

Small size represents a failure of growth, which in the fetus is potentially limited by the availability of nutrients. Therefore, it has been suggested that diet and nutrition might be the major factors which determine the programming of metabolic function. However, because epidemiological studies do not of themselves provide proof positive of causality, there has been some scepticism that the observations, while interesting, should not be taken to imply a causal relationship between maternal diet during pregnancy and the later programming of metabolic function in her offspring. There is considerable literature to show that severe nutritional deprivation in animals leads to irreversible growth failure in the offspring (McCance & Widdowson, 1974). It has been less clear whether more modest variation in diet, as seen amongst women who give birth to babies of very different size, can possibly underlie such profound effects. However, more recent evidence from animal studies show that even modest dietary manipulations during pregnancy of the macronutrient and micronutrient intake within the range normally consumed, can lead to reproducible changes in a wide range of functions in the offspring.

These effects are specific and include increased blood pressure, glucose intolerance, changes in appetite control, central fat deposition, immune dysfunction, changes in inflammatory responses and behavioural alterations (Jackson *et al.*, 1996). Even very short periods of exposure to quite modest dietary manipulations during early pregnancy can have profound effects, leading to changes in the structure and expression of specific genes related to intermediary metabolism and cellular control. One possible underlying change might be that the placental barrier to maternal glucocorticoids is impaired by nutritional insult and the fetus is overexposed to maternal glucocorticoids which modulate the development of its glucocorticoid sensitive systems. Thus, the availability of nutrients creates a particular hormonal milieu, and the two interact to induce an effect by modulating the expression of genes critical for developmental processes (Wootton & Jackson, 1996). A direct effect is exerted upon the critical set of the main centres in the hypothalamus which integrate metabolism, control behaviour and determine the function of cells and tissues.

The fetus carries its 'blueprint' for development in its genes, but to realise this potential requires an adequate supply and delivery of nutrients (oxygen, water, energy, substrates and cofactors) sufficient to meet the demand. Growth and development are structured in time and therefore the pattern of demand varies as pregnancy advances, varying the pattern which the mother has to provide for her fetus at each stage of pregnancy. If the mother were solely dependent upon her dietary intake to meet the changing nutrient needs of her fetus, this would be a very high risk strategy. Adequate reserves are essential for a successful outcome. For women who are generally well nourished, differences in dietary intake account for 5% of the variability in birth weight. Taller women have heavier babies. Height is of importance as a measure of ability of the mother to provide an optimal nutritional environment for her unborn baby. Low body weight before becoming pregnant leads to reduced birth weight, which can in part be offset by greater weight gain during pregnancy. There is a special risk of poorer fetal growth in women who are short and fat than in women who are taller and fat, or short and of appropriate weight. Those women who become pregnant while still in their teenage years, at a time when they are still growing, face the special problem of there being competition between providing enough nutrients for the continuing growth of the mother and the needs of the baby. They are very likely to have smaller babies.

During the first weeks of pregnancy the organ systems of the embryo are developing. The nutritional status of a woman before she becomes pregnant determines the quality of the nutrient environment of the early embryo before the placenta has formed and developed any function. The ability of the mother to provide sufficient nutrients to the placenta once it has formed determines the rate at which the fetus is able to grow and develop. The rate at which protein is synthesised in the mother is related to her height and her visceral mass, and in turn protein synthesis around 18 weeks gestation is closely related to newborn length. The fetus requires a particular mix of nutrients, which to a large extent is dependent upon metabolic transformation in the mother, which in turn requires an adequate micronutrient status.

During the third trimester about half of fetal weight gain is adipose tissue and nearly half the variability in birth weight is accounted for by differences in the adipose tissue content of the newborn. In the first part of pregnancy fat accumulates in the mother's tissues to be used to meet the needs of the baby as the demand increases during the last 10 weeks of pregnancy. At this time the circulating lipids in the mother increase to very high levels and the effective mobilisation of maternal lipid and its availability across the placenta is determined by the mother's ability to regulate her intermediary disposal of dietary and endogenous lipid. As well as providing large amounts of lipid for the unborn baby, the mother also has to provide lipid of a suitable quality. Lipid is required for the normal structure of all the membranes in the cells which are being formed. This is especially true for the developing brain, where myelination is critically dependent upon adequate provision of n-3 fatty acids. It would be very difficult to meet the considerable demand over a short period of time from the diet alone and therefore adequate reserves laid down before pregnancy or during the early weeks of pregnancy become very important. The interconversion of specific fatty acids is also important, and for this to take place at a suitable rate requires that the micronutrient status of the mother is optimal. Thus in animal studies, for example, poor iron status interferes with the normal interconversion of essential fatty acids and impairs myelination of the brain leading to poorer learning and memory. Iron status itself is influenced by a range of other factors beyond simple consumption, such as infection, overall quality of the diet, and an adequate intake of other micronutrients.

Dietary guidelines for pregnancy

These complex interactions make it very difficult to implicate one factor as being especially important compared with any other. Dietary guidelines for pregnancy should place an emphasis upon women being in a good nutritional state at the time of conception. Once a pregnancy has been established, guidelines should emphasise the need to consume a varied balanced diet against the background of reasonable activity and adequate rest.

There are a number of factors which interact with diet and exert an adverse effect upon pregnancy, most importantly smoking and alcohol consumption, infections, and pregnancy at a young age. Women who smoke have babies which are 200 g lighter on average. This adverse effect is in part the direct result of toxicity, but may also be induced in part through diet. In general people who smoke consume a diet which is less healthy, and probably have an increased need for adequate micronutrients to provide antioxidant and anti-inflammatory protection. Low grade infection in the mother, leading to chronic inflammation, is quite common in pregnancy and increases the risk to the fetus. Apart from direct toxic effects, inflammation reduces the availability of nutrients to the fetus as the mother diverts available resource to cope with the underlying inflammatory processes.

Competition for nutrients between the mother and the fetus is most likely to reach serious proportions in women who become pregnant at a time when they have not yet completed their own growth. Thus the baby of a teenager will be about 200 g lighter than the baby of a similar women in her twenties. A teenage pregnancy is a direct cause of poor fetal growth. Their babies are 70% more likely to be born small, either through pre-maturity or poor growth. It has been estimated that to have a baby of equivalent weight an adolescent has to gain an extra 4 kg during preg-nancy, is more likely to gain excess fat, and finds it more difficult to lose the fat after the baby has been born. There is a clear difference in birth weight between different ethnic groups which cannot be explained simply by differences in social conditions. In particular babies of mothers from the Indian subcontinent are likely to be up to 400 g lighter.

Thus, the effective nutritional preparation for pregnancy starts many years before conception. The growth of all young women and men is important in this regard, and the future health of the population is critically related to the nutritional well-being of children from an early age. Although single factors can be identified which exert a particularly adverse effect, there are many complex inter-relationships. Not engaging in damaging beha-viour is clearly of importance, and refraining from smoking, limiting alcohol consumption and taking regular exercise can be of considerable benefit. Dietary guidelines for pregnancy should place emphasis on women being in a good nutritional state at the time of conception. Once a pregnancy has been established, guidelines should emphasise the need to consume a varied and balanced diet against the background of reasonable activity and adequate rest. Within this dietary variety there is the need to ensure that the consumption of all micronutrients is maximised, preferably through the consumption of generous amounts of fresh fruit and vegetables. Considerable emphasis should be placed on the benefit to the baby of delaying the first pregnancy until after the mother's twentieth birthday.

References

Barker, D.J.P. (1998) *Mothers, Babies and Health in Later Life*. Churchill Livingstone, Edinburgh.

Jackson, A.A. (1999) Perinatal nutrition: the impact on postnatal growth and development. In: *Pediatrics and Perinatology* (eds P.D. Gluckman & M.A. Heymann), pp. 298–303. Arnold, London.

Jackson, A.A., Langley-Evans, S.C. & McCarthy, H.D. (1996) Nutritional influences in early life upon obesity and body proportions. In: *The Origins and Consequence of Obesity* (eds D.J. Chadwick & G. Cardew), pp. 118–37. John Wiley & Sons, Chichester.

McCance, R.A. & Widdowson, E.M. (1974) The determinants of growth and form. *Proc. Roy. Soc.*, **185**, 1–17.

Wootton, S.A. & Jackson, A.A. (1996) Influence of under-nutrition in early life on growth, body composition and metabolic competence. In: *Long Term Consequences of Early Environment Growth: development and the lifespan developmental perspective* (eds C.J.K. Henry & S.J. Ulijaszek), pp. 109–23. Cambridge University Press, Cambridge.

11

PLANT BASED DIETS: FINDINGS FROM THE OXFORD VEGETARIAN STUDY AND OTHER PROSPECTIVE STUDIES OF VEGETARIANS

TIMOTHY J. KEY, PAUL N. APPLEBY, NAOMI E. ALLEN,
GWYNETH K. DAVEY, MARGARET THOROGOOD AND JIM I. MANN

Introduction

Interest in plant based diets is increasing, because this type of diet may offer protection against some of the chronic diseases common in Western countries. It can also have major advantages in terms of efficient land use, and is an ethical preference for many people. Knowledge of the nutritional implications of a plant-based diet is substantial, but data on the long-term health effects of this type of diet are more limited. In the early 1980s researchers in Oxford established a prospective cohort study of 11 000 subjects to examine the long-term health of vegetarians in the UK. Results have been published from this study on the health characteristics of the subjects, focusing particularly on lipid levels, and the mortality rates after 12–13 years of follow up, focusing on all-cause mortality and deaths from ischaemic heart disease (IHD) (Thorogood, *et al.*, 1987, 1990, 1994; Mann *et al.*, 1997). In this chapter we describe the main findings from this cohort, present some additional data from a second prospective study of 58 000 subjects recently established in Oxford (a component of EPIC, the European Prospective Investigation into Cancer and Nutrition (Riboli & Kaaks, 1997)), and summarise the results from other major prospective studies of vegetarians.

Diet: foods and nutrients

By definition, vegetarians eat no meat or fish, and the macronutrients supplied by these foods in an omnivorous diet are supplied by plant foods and also, for lacto-ovovegetarians, by dairy products and eggs. Meat, and to a lesser extent fish, are rich in energy, protein and fat; vegetarians typically replace animal sources of these macronutrients by consuming more cereals, legumes, nuts and vegetable oils than omnivores. Vegetarians usually also consume more fruits and vegetables than omnivores, although these foods are not major sources of energy or other macronutrients and therefore do not replace meat and fish in the diet.

The food intake pattern of vegetarians produces a nutrient intake pattern with some important differences from the nutrient intake of omnivores. In the Oxford Vegetarian Study, vegetarians were observed to consume less protein and more carbohydrate and dietary fibre than meat eaters. Total fat intake was similar in vegetarians and meat eaters, but the composition of the fat differed, with vegetarians having a higher ratio of polyunsaturated to saturated fatty acids, and also a lower intake of cholesterol (Thorogood *et al.*, 1990). Similar results have been observed among the vegetarians recruited more recently into the Oxford EPIC study (Allen *et al.*, 2000 and unpublished data).

Body mass index

One of the most consistent observations in relation to diet and body mass index (BMI) is that Western vegetarians tend to have a lower BMI than Western non-vegetarians. In an analysis of data for 5300 non-smokers in the Oxford Vegetarian Study, mean BMI was lower in non-meat eaters than in meat eaters in all age groups for both men and women (Appleby *et al.*, 1998). Overall age-adjusted mean BMIs in kg m^{-2} were 23.2 and 22.1 for male meat eaters and non-meat eaters respectively ($P<0.0001$), and 22.3 and 21.3 for female meat eaters and non-meat eaters respectively ($P<0.0001$). Examination of other dietary and lifestyle factors showed that, as well as meat consumption, dietary fibre intake, animal fat intake, social class and previous smoking were all independently associated with BMI in both men and women. BMI was also independently associated with alcohol consumption in men and with parity in women. After adjusting for these factors the differences in age-adjusted mean BMI between meat eaters and non-meat eaters were reduced by 36% in men and 31% in women. Thus a higher intake of dietary fibre, a lower intake of animal fat, and in men a lower intake of alcohol, account for some but not all of the difference in BMI between vegetarians and non-vegetarians.

Similar results were obtained from an analysis of BMI by dietary group in the Oxford cohort of the EPIC study (Key & Davey 1996; Key *et al.*, 1999a). Mean BMI was about 1 kg m^{-2} lower among vegetarians than among meat eaters in both men and women, and this corresponded to a substantially lower prevalence of obesity among the vegetarians.

Plasma lipids

Plasma lipids and diet groups

Concentrations of total cholesterol and various lipoprotein fractions were compared in four diet groups in the Oxford Vegetarian Study: vegans, vegetarians, fish eaters (who did not eat meat), and meat eaters (Thorogood *et al.*, 1987). Mean total cholesterol concentrations, adjusted for age and sex, were 4.29, 4.88, 5.01, and 5.31 mmol l^{-1} for vegans, vegetarians, fish eaters and meat eaters respectively. These differences in total cholesterol were largely due to differences in LDL-cholesterol, since HDL-cholesterol did not differ between vegans, vegetarians and meat eaters (although HDL-cholesterol was about 5% higher in the fish eaters than in the other dietary groups). On the basis of these results it was predicted that the incidence of ischaemic heart disease might be 24% lower in lifelong vegetarians, and 57% lower in lifelong vegans, than in meat eaters.

Similar differences in cholesterol have also been observed in the subjects recruited during the 1990s into the Oxford component of the EPIC study. Among 696 men, the mean total cholesterol concentrations were 4.08, 4.55 and 4.94 mmol l^{-1} in vegans, vegetarians and meat eaters respectively (Allen *et al.*, 2000). Among 1097 women, mean total cholesterol concentrations were 3.55, 3.85 and 4.18 mmol l-1 in premenopausal vegans, vegetarians and meat eaters, and 4.55, 5.01 and 5.36 in postmenopausal vegans, vegetarians and meat eaters respectively (Thomas *et al.*, 1999). As in the Oxford Vegetarian Study, these differences in total cholesterol were due to differences in LDL-cholesterol, and HDL-cholesterol did not differ between women in the three dietary groups (Thomas *et al.*, 1999). (Cholesterol subfractions have not been assayed among the men in this study).

Plasma lipids and nutrient intake

The relationship between plasma lipids and nutrient intake was examined by Thorogood *et al.* (1990). Cholesterol concentrations in 208 subjects matched for age and sex were analysed in relation to nutrient intakes derived from the analysis of four-day food diaries. Total cholesterol concentration was positively correlated with the Keys score (partial $r = 0.37$; $P<0.001$, controlling for age, sex and BMI). HDL-cholesterol concentration was positively associated with dietary cholesterol (partial $r = 0.13$; $P<0.05$), and with alcohol intake as a percentage of total energy (partial $r = 0.26$; $P<0.001$). It was concluded that the nature rather than the quantity of dietary fat is an important determinant of plasma cholesterol concentration, and that the individuals in this study with a low serum cholesterol level tend to select a fat-modified, rather than a low fat diet. The relatively low serum total cholesterol concentration of vegetarians is probably explained by their relatively low intake of saturated fat and cholesterol, and their relatively high intake of polyunsaturated fat.

Plasma lipids, foods and lifestyle

The effects of dietary, lifestyle and physical factors on serum concentrations of total and HDL-cholesterol were further investigated by Appleby *et al.* (1995). In this analysis, the emphasis was on individual foods rather than on nutrients, and stepwise multiple linear regression was used to determine which foods, lifestyle and physical factors were associated with cholesterol concentration. Meat and cheese consumption were positively associated, and dietary fibre intake inversely associated, with total cholesterol concentration in both men and women. Other factors positively associated with total cholesterol concentration were smoking in men, and the use of saturated spreading fats and (unexpectedly) tomato consumption in women, while height in men was inversely associated with total cholesterol concentration. In contrast, none of the dietary factors investigated had a significant effect on HDL-cholesterol concentration (except for a positive association with the use of saturated spreading fats in women). However, HDL-cholesterol concentration was positively associated with alcohol intake and inversely associated with BMI. The results provided further evidence of the cholesterol-lowering effect of diets with limited use of meat and cheese and with a high fibre content.

Hormones

Sex hormone and growth factor concentrations in men

Sex hormones, in particular testosterone, may play a key role in the aetiology of prostate cancer, and there is substantial interest in the possible effects of dietary factors on sex hormone metabolism. To test the hypothesis that a vegan diet may reduce hormone levels in men, concentrations of total testosterone, free testosterone, total oestradiol and sex hormone binding globulin (SHBG) were determined in 51 vegan and 57 meat-eating men in the Oxford Vegetarian Study (Key *et al.*, 1990). No significant differences in the mean concentrations of sex hormones were found, although SHBG concentration was 23% higher among the vegans compared to the meat eaters (P = 0.001). Later, a much larger study based on the Oxford EPIC cohort confirmed that there were no significant differences in free testosterone levels between 233 vegans, 237 vegetarians and 226 meat eaters, although again SHBG levels were significantly higher among vegan men than in vegetarians or meat eaters (Allen *et al.*, 2000). A new finding from this study was that the mean concentration of insulin-like growth factor-I (IGF-I), also thought to be a risk factor for prostate cancer, was 9% lower among vegan men compared with vegetarians and meat eaters (*P* = 0.002; Allen *et al.*, 2000).

Sex hormone concentrations in women

In an investigation of the hormonal factors thought to influence breast cancer risk, concentrations of plasma oestradiol and SHBG were determined among 640 premenopausal women and 457 postmenopausal women from different dietary groups (Thomas *et al.*, 1999). This study found no significant differences in the mean oestradiol or SHBG concentrations between vegans, vegetarians or meat eaters, among either the premenopausal or postmenopausal women. No study has thus far investigated the differences in IGF-I concentration among female meat eaters and non-meat eaters.

Mortality

Mortality by diet group

Mortality in the Oxford Vegetarian Study was first studied after an average of 12 years follow-up (Thorogood *et al.*, 1994). Subjects were divided into meat eaters (who ate meat at least once a week) and non-meat eaters (all others) most of whom were vegetarian or vegan. Standardised mortality ratios (SMRs) were calculated for all causes of death, ischaemic heart disease, and all malignant neoplasms, based on 404 deaths before age 80. As expected, the death rate in the whole cohort was significantly lower than in the reference population of England and Wales (standardised mortality ratios and 95% confidence intervals were: 0.46 (0.42–0.51) for all causes of death, 0.38 (0.30–0.46) for ischaemic heart disease, and 0.62

(0.53–0.73) for all malignant neoplasms). The relatively low death rates were attributed to the 'healthy volunteer effect' and the fact that subjects were recruited from a health-conscious sector of the population.

Within the cohort, death rates were lower in the non-meat eaters than the meat eaters for all three end points examined. The results were similar for men and women, and after restricting the analysis to subjects who had never smoked. However, when the first five years of follow-up were excluded from the analysis, the death rate ratios became closer to unity and were not statistically significant. Further examination of the association of a vegetarian diet with mortality was therefore planned by conducting a pooled analysis of the world-wide data (see below).

Mortality in relation to foods and animal fats

The effects of various dietary factors on mortality from ischaemic heart disease and from all causes of death in the Oxford Vegetarian Study were examined by Mann *et al.* (1997). Subjects were grouped not just according to their diet but also by their consumption of various foods, and according to their estimated intake of total fat, saturated fat and dietary cholesterol, and by their estimated dietary fibre intake. The main analysis was restricted to subjects with no cardiovascular disease or diabetes at recruitment. All death rate ratios were adjusted for age, sex, smoking and social class. The analysis included a total of 525 deaths before age 80 in an average of 13.3 years of follow-up, of which 392 deaths were in subjects with no pre-existing disease at recruitment, including 64 deaths from ischaemic heart disease. The most striking result from the analysis was the strong positive association between increasing consumption of animal fats and ischaemic heart disease mortality. Death rate ratios and 95% confidence intervals for the highest third of intake compared with the lowest third were 3.29 (1.50–7.21) for total animal fat, 2.77 (1.25–6.13) for saturated animal fat, and 3.53 (1.57–7.96) for dietary cholesterol. In contrast, no protective effects were noted for dietary fibre, fish or alcohol consumption. The effects of individual foods on all-cause mortality were generally indeterminate, although there was a suggestion of an inverse association with nut consumption and a U-shaped relationship with the consumption of both eggs and milk.

Pooled analysis of the world-wide data on mortality in vegetarians

The Oxford Vegetarian Study cohort of 11 000 subjects is too small to produce precise estimates of mortality rates, particularly for single causes of death such as specific cancers. We therefore decided to pool the original data from the Oxford Vegetarian Study with data from four other cohort studies which also included substantial proportions (around 40%) of vegetarians; we were particularly interested in confirming the reduction in mortality from ischaemic heart disease in vegetarians observed in the Oxford Vegetarian Study, and also in examining the hypothesis that vegetarians might have a relatively low mortality from colorectal cancer. Data were available for 76 000 subjects (including 28 000 vegetarians) among whom there were 8300 deaths before age 90 during follow-up. Results were adjusted for age, sex and smoking (Key *et al.*, 1998, 1999b).

Ischaemic heart disease

In the pooled analysis of the world-wide data on mortality in vegetarians, there were 2300 deaths from ischaemic heart disease. The mortality from ischaemic heart disease was 24% lower in vegetarians than in non-vegetarians (death rate ratio: 0.76, 95% CI 0.62-0.94, *P*<0.01). The reduction was greatest for deaths at younger ages, with a 45% reduction (95% CI 15% to 65%) for deaths below age 65. The reduction in mortality appeared to be confined to those who had been vegetarian for more than 5 years.

Colorectal cancer

Contrary to our hypothesis, there was no significant difference in colorectal cancer mortality between vegetarians and non-vegetarians (death rate ratio: 0.99, 95% CI 0.77-1.27, based on 278 deaths). This result does not completely exclude some effect of meat on the development of colorectal cancer, but does imply that colorectal cancer rates are not particularly low in vegetarians and that dietary factors other than meat may explain the large variation in the risks of colorectal cancer between different populations.

Other causes of death

There were no significant differences in mortality for any of the other causes of death studied. Death rate ratios for vegetarians compared with non-vegetarians were 1.02 (95% CI 0.64-1.62) for stomach cancer, 0.84 (0.59-1.18) for lung cancer, 0.95 (0.55-1.63) for female breast cancer, 0.91 (0.60-1.39) for prostate cancer, 0.93 (0.74-1.17) for cerebrovascular disease, and 0.95 (0.82-1.11) for all causes of death combined.

Conclusions

The Western vegetarians who have participated in the Oxford Vegetarian Study and in the other prospective studies appear to enjoy good health. They have relatively low serum cholesterol concentrations and a low prevalence of obesity, and their mortality rates are substantially lower than the national averages. When compared with non-vegetarians who have an otherwise similar lifestyle, vegetarians have a lower mortality from ischaemic heart disease, which might be explained by their low serum cholesterol concentrations. Relatively few data are available for other causes of death including the common cancers, and so far no differences in cancer rates between vegetarians and comparable non-vegetarians have been established. A paper describing updated follow-up of the Oxford Vegetarian Study will be published shortly, and over the next few years further data on the long-term health consequences of plant-based diets will become available from the Oxford component of EPIC and from other studies.

Acknowledgements

Thanks are due to all of the participants in the Oxford Vegetarian Study and the EPIC Study, and to the scientists who have assisted with the analysis of data arising from these studies. These studies have been supported by the Imperial Cancer Research Fund, the Cancer Research Campaign, and the Europe Against Cancer Programme of the Commission of the European Communities.

References

Allen, N.E., Appleby, P.N., Davey, G.K. & Key, T.J. (2000) Hormones and diet: low insulin-like growth factor-I but normal bioavailable androgens in vegan men. *Br. J. Cancer*, **83**, 95–7.

Appleby, P.N., Thorogood, M., McPherson, K. & Mann, J.I. (1995) Associations between plasma lipid concentrations and dietary, lifestyle and physical factors in the Oxford Vegetarian Study. *J. Human Nutr. Dietetics*, **8**, 305–14.

Appleby, P.N., Thorogood, M., Mann, J.I. & Key, T.J. (1998) Low BMI in non-meat eaters: the possible roles of animal fat, dietary fibre and alcohol. *Int. J. Obes.*, **22**, 454–60.

Key, T.J.A., Roe, L., Thorogood, M., Moore, J.W., Clark, G.G. & Wang, D.Y. (1990) Testosterone, sex hormone-binding globulin, calculated free testosterone, and estradiol in male vegans and omnivores. *Br. J. Nutr.*, **64**, 111–19.

Key, T.J. & Davey, G.K. (1996) Prevalence of obesity is low in people who do not eat meat. *BMJ*, **313**, 816–17.

Key, T.J., Fraser, G.E., Thorogood, M., Appleby, P.N., Beral, V., Reeves, G. Burr, M.L., Chang-Claude, J., Frentzel-Beyme, R., Kuzma, J.W., Mann, J. & McPherson, K. (1998) Mortality in vegetarians and non-vegetarians: a collaborative analysis of 8300 deaths among 76000 men and women in five prospective studies. *Public Health Nutrition*, **1**, 33–41.

Key, T.J., Davey, G.K. & Appleby, P.N. (1999a) Health benefits of a vegetarian diet. *Proc. Nutr. Soc.*, **58**, 271–5.

Key, T.J.A., Fraser, G.E., Thorogood, M., Appleby, P.N., Beral, V., Reeves, G., Burr, M.L., Chang-Claude, J., Frentzel-Beyme, R., Kuzma, J.W., Mann, J. & McPherson, K. (1999b) Mortality in vegetarians: detailed findings from a collaborative analysis of five prospective studies. *Am. J. Clin. Nutr.*, **70**, 516S–24S.

Mann, J.I., Appleby, P.N., Key, T.J.A. & Thorogood M. (1997) Dietary determinants of ischaemic heart disease in health-conscious individuals. *Heart*, **78**, 450–55.

Riboli, E. & Kaaks, R. (1997) The EPIC Project: rationale and study design. *Int. J. Epidemiol.*, **26**, S6–14.

Thomas, H.V., Davey, G.K. & Key, T.J. (1999) Oestradiol and sex hormone-binding globulin in premenopausal and post-menopausal meat eaters, vegetarians and vegans. *Br. J. Cancer*, **80**, 1470–75.

Thorogood, M., Carter, R., Benfield, L., McPherson, K. & Mann J.I. (1987) Plasma lipids and lipoprotein cholesterol concentrations in people with different diets in Britain. *BMJ*, **295**, 351–3.

Thorogood, M., Roe, L., McPherson, K. & Mann, J. (1990) Dietary intake and plasma lipid levels: lessons from a study of the diet of health conscious groups. *BMJ*, **300**, 1297–1301.

Thorogood, M., Mann, J., Appleby, P. & McPherson, K. (1994) Risk of death from cancer and ischaemic heart disease in meat and non-meat eaters. *BMJ*, **308**, 1667–71.

12

REVIEW OF DIET AND CANCER: WHAT IS THE EVIDENCE?

MICHAEL HILL

The success of the anti-smoking campaigns in many European, North American and Oceanic countries (Peto *et al.*, 2000) shows that cancer prevention can work. Diet is as important a cause of cancer as is smoking (Wynder & Gori, 1977; Doll & Peto, 1981), and so in principle we should be able to achieve the same level of success. However, whereas there are only health benefits from giving up smoking, there is a risk-benefit equation for most dietary change. This often leads to controversy, an inconsistent message, and consequent cynicism amongst the general public. If we hope to decrease the numbers of diet-related cancers we must do as those in the anti-smoking campaign have done. We must find a consistent message, backed by solid evidence.

For historical reasons, much of the early work on cancer prevention was devoted to identifying 'causes' and then trying to eliminate them. This is the 'infectious disease model'. However, the evidence for this, in the case of diet-related cancers, is in all cases very weak and controversial. In contrast, we know much more about foods that help us to defend against cancer, such as a high intake of fruit, vegetables and whole grain cereals, together with maintenance of a 'healthy' body weight. The evidence suggests that we should abandon the infectious disease model of diet-related cancers in favour of a 'nutrient deficiency model'. For this reason, most organisations concerned with cancer prevention now advise that to reduce the risk of cancer we should eat a diet rich in fruit, vegetables and whole grain cereals, and avoid overweight by taking plenty of exercise.

Avoid overweight

There is firm evidence that overweight is a risk factor for cancers at many
sites in the body, including the colon and prostate for men, and the colon,
breast, endometrium, ovary and gall bladder for women (reviewed by Hill,
1995). Overweight is a consequence of an excess of energy intake over
energy expenditure. However, the evidence does not support excess
energy intake as the risk factor for cancer (DoH, 1998). In contrast there is
a growing body of evidence that lack of exercise is a risk factor for all of
the cancers associated with overweight (reviewed by Hill, 2001).

Whereas there is an abundance of quantitative evidence that exercise
protects against heart disease, the evidence with respect to cancer risk is
qualitative rather than quantitative. In consequence, the provisional
recommendations tend to be to take 2–3 hours of brisk exercise per week.

Eat plenty of fruit and vegetables

The evidence from reviews of case-control studies that a diet rich in fruit
and vegetables is associated with a decreased risk of cancer at many sites is
overwhelming, and was reviewed elsewhere by Hill (1995, 2001). In
general, the evidence in favour of fruits is strongest for cancers of the
respiratory tract and the upper digestive tract. The evidence for vegetables being protective is strongest for cancers of the lower digestive tract.

Here the evidence is more quantitative, and supports the recommendation that we should eat at least five portions per day of fruit and vegetables. A 'portion' is approximately 100 g. In the North Italian studies (La
Vecchia & Tavani, 1998) there was a strong dose-response relationship
between intake of both fruits and vegetables and risk of cancer at a wide
range of sites. They calculated that each additional portion of fruit and
vegetable gives a 10% reduction in cancer risk. No individual fruit or
vegetable appears to be any better than the others; they are all good.
However, the evidence from the North Italian study was that the protection was increased by maximising the range of different fruits and
vegetables consumed.

Whole grain cereals

There is similar evidence that whole grain cereals protect against cancer
of the colon and breast, and perhaps against a wide range of sites (Jacobs
et al., 1996; Hill, 1997; La Vecchia & Chatenoud, 1998). The wide range of

sites suggests that the protection does not come entirely from the dietary fibre component.

The evidence suggests that the diet should contain enough whole grain cereal to supply at least 16 g of cereal fibre. A standard portion of high fibre breakfast cereal supplies about 10 g, and so starting the day with a high fibre breakfast cereal is the best way to reach the target. If you have a glass of fruit juice with it, and perhaps finish with a banana, this would also supply the first two of your 'five-a-day'.

Other foods

The evidence for other foods or nutrients is much less firm. The evidence, for example, that fish consumption protects against colorectal and breast cancer is equivocal. If fish are protective it is not clear whether the protection comes from the pufa, or from the antioxidants there to protect the pufa.

Olive oil is protective in some studies, but it is not certain whether it is the olive oil or the salad that it is eaten with that provides the protection. If it is the olive oil, is the protection from the mufa? Or does it come the host of antioxidants present in the olive oil to protect the unsaturated fatty acid from oxidation?

A range of micronutrients has been cited, but the evidence is inconclusive for all of them.

Conclusions

We are in a position to deliver a positive message on diet and cancer prevention that we can all agree on, and that has been outlined above. It is a set of recommendations for cancer in general, not just for a particular high-profile site (such as breast cancer or colon cancer). This is important. Some cancers (such as the breast, colon and prostate) are associated with a 'rich' diet, while some (such as the stomach, oesophagus and liver) are associated with 'poor' diets; there is no value in a diet which reduces the risk of cancer at one site if it promotes cancer at another!

If we all stress this common message, then we can hope that eventually the public will conclude that we have now reached agreement and will listen to us. If, on the other hand, we indulge our egos by continuing to call press conferences to stress the perils (or magical properties) of a particular food, or if we over-hype a particular study with unusual results, then of course the public will remain confused and will ignore us.

References

DoH (1998) *Nutritional aspects of the development of cancer.* The Stationery Office, London.

Doll, R. & Peto, R. (1981) The causes of cancer; quantitative estimates of avoidable risk of cancer in the United States. *JNCI,* **66**, 1191-1308.

Hill, M.J. (1995) Diet and cancer; a review of the scientific evidence. *Eur. J. Cancer Prev.,* **4** (suppl. 2), 3-42.

Hill, M.J. (1997) Cereals, cereal fibre and colorectal cancer risk; a review of the epidemiological literature. *Eur. J. Cancer Prev.,* **6**, 219-25.

Hill, M.J. (2001) ECP dietary advice on cancer prevention. *Eur. J. Cancer Prev.,* **10**, (in press).

Jacobs, D.R., Slavin, J. & Marquardt, L. (1996) Whole grain intake and cancer; a review of the literature. *Nutr. Cancer,* **24**, 221-9.

La Vecchia, C. & Chatenoud, L. (1998) Fibres, whole grain foods and breast and other cancers. *Eur. J. Cancer Prev.,* **7** (suppl. 2), s25-8.

La Vecchia, C. & Tavani, A. (1998) Fruit and vegetables and human cancer. *Eur. J. Cancer Prev.,* **7**, 3-8.

Peto, R., Darby, S, Deo H., Silcockx, P., Whitley, E. & Doll, R. (2000) Smoking, smoking cessation and lung cancer in the UK since 1950; combination of national statistics with two case-control studies. *BMJ,* **321**, 323-9.

Wynder, E. & Gori, G. (1977) Contribution of the environment to cancer incidence; an epidemiological exercise. *JNCI,* **58**, 825-32.

13

MICRONUTRIENTS, PHYTOPROTECTANTS AND MECHANISMS OF ANTICANCER ACTIVITY

IAN T. JOHNSON

Introduction

Throughout history, the principal causes of death in most human populations have been infant mortality, infectious disease and the chronic conditions of old age – principally cancer, heart disease and stroke. Because deaths from the first two causes tend to decline dramatically with increasing prosperity, cancer and cardiovascular disease now inevitably cause a growing proportion of deaths in industrialised countries. However even in the nineteenth century, Tanchou proposed that urban societies were characterised by increasing rates of cancer (Tanchou, 1843), and careful international studies of age-corrected rates for cancer continue to support this view. Doll and Peto estimated that diet was responsible for approximately 35% of cancers in the West (Doll & Peto, 1981), and more recently the World Cancer Research Fund has confirmed the central importance of diet as a major determinant of many forms of cancer across the globe (World Cancer Research Fund, 1997).

In principle, diet may influence the incidence of cancer in a population via exposure to food-borne carcinogens, or by providing protective factors. With the possible exceptions of alcohol and mutagens derived from cooked meat, the levels of known carcinogens in food appear too low to account for the observed levels of human disease (Lutz & Schlatter, 1992). However, a large body of epidemiological evidence has accumulated in favour of the protective effects of plant foods (Block *et al.*,1992). This chapter briefly reviews the role of recognised micronutrients, and the so-called 'phytoprotectants', secondary plant metabolites with biological activity in human metabolism.

Mechanisms of action

Much of the fundamental work upon which our current understanding of human cancer rests has been developed with the aid of animal models. Carcinogenesis is a prolonged, multistage process during which the tumour cells gradually acquire mutations in key genes regulating cellular proliferation and differentiation (Bodmer, 1994), and which usually occupies a large proportion of an individual's life span. Because of this complexity and long duration, there are many critical steps where food components may interact so as to delay or even reverse the process. To simplify matters, dietary anticarcinogens can be classified as blocking agents, which operate during the initiation phase of carcinogenesis, and suppressing agents, which delay or reverse tumour promotion at a later stage (Wattenburg, 1990). Blocking substances prevent DNA damage, for example by quenching reactive oxygen species of detoxifying mutagenic chemicals. Phase I and Phase II biotransformation enzymes, which are expressed strongly in the gastrointestinal mucosa and in the liver, act as a first line of defence against toxic substances in the environment, and certain dietary constituents can inhibit Phase I enzymes and others enhance Phase II activity, thus minimising the activation of carcinogens and increasing their excretion.

Experimental animal studies have also shown that some substances can inhibit the appearance of tumours, even when given days or weeks after exposure to a chemical carcinogen (Wattenburg, 1990). In these circumstances the mechanism of action must be due to some reduction in the rate at which initiated cells develop into tumours, rather than to any reduction in DNA damage. Tumour suppression is poorly understood, but it probably involves inhibition of cell proliferation, increased cellular differentiation, and apoptosis, whereby cells bearing mutations are eliminated entirely from the tissue (Johnson *et al.*, 1994).

Dietary components

The World Cancer Research Fund report on diet and cancer (Lutz & Schlatter, 1992) recommended that individuals should consume nutritionally adequate and varied diets based predominantly on fruits, vegetables, pulses and minimally processed starchy foods. Excess weight, defined as body mass index in excess of 25, is associated with a rise in the relative risk of most cancers, and obesity is particularly associated with cancers of the breast and endometrium. For these reasons the report recommended that BMI should be maintained between 18.5 and 25. The recommendation to consume a variety of fruits and vegetables reflects the growing evidence that plant foods contain protective factors, including both micronutrients and phytoprotectants.

Antioxidant nutrients

Mutations can occur as a result of oxidative damage to DNA caused by free-radicals generated as a side effect of aerobic metabolism (Halliwell, 1994). Plant and animal cells defend themselves against these effects by deploying antioxidants to trap or quench free-radicals and hence arrest their damaging reactions. Many of those in the human body are derived from the diet. The theory that free-radicals are a major cause of human cancer, and that the risk of disease can be reduced by increased consumption of food-borne antioxidants, has prompted enormous interest in food-borne antioxidants, such as the nutrients, vitamins A, C and E. Nevertheless the role of mutagenesis due to oxygen free-radicals in the pathogenesis of human cancers in well-nourished populations remains unproven, and attempts to prevent cancer by intervention with high doses of antioxidant vitamins have been largely unsuccessful (Albanes *et al.*, 1995).

Carotenoids

Another group of phytochemicals that are of interest in this context are the carotenoids, of which approximately 500 have been identified in vegetables and fruits used as human foods. The vast majority occur at low concentrations and are probably of little biological significance, but ß-carotene is classified as nutrient because it is the precursor for vitamin A. Others, including lycopene and lutein, are abundant in tomatoes and coloured vegetables (Khachik *et al.*, 1995). The molecular structure of the carotenoids includes an extended chain of double bonds, which enables them to function as antioxidants. Carotenoids are released from plant foods in the small intestine and absorbed in conjunction with dietary fat. ß-Carotene occurs in plasma in direct proportion to dietary intake of fruits and vegetables. There is good epidemiological evidence for an inverse association between intake of carotenoids and cancers of the lung and bowel, and one possible explanation for this is that they protect these tissues against oxidative damage. However, intervention trials with ß-carotene have proved disappointing (Greenberg *et al.*, 1994; Albanes *et al.*, 1995), and the carotenoids may simply be acting as biomarkers of fruit and vegetable consumption.

Folates

Naturally occurring folates originate from green plants and yeast cells, and are also plentiful in liver and kidney. They and their derivatives act as coenzymes in reactions involving transfer of single carbon groups during the synthesis of amino acids and DNA. Folate deficient diets are associated with increased risk of hepatic cancer in animal models. The precise relationship between folate metabolism and carcinogenesis is unclear, but the link may lie in the role of folate coenzymes in the control of DNA methylation. Ma *et al.* (1997) explored the relationship between risk of colorectal carcinoma and a common mutation affecting the activity of the enzyme 5,10-methylenetetrahydrofolate, reductase in a large cohort study. The presence of a homozygous mutation was shown to reduce the risk of colorectal cancer in men with adequate folate levels, but the protection was absent in men with low overall folate status. One possible explanation for this effect is that low levels of MTHFR expression shunt folates into DNA synthesis, thereby helping to maintain normal patterns of DNA methylation. There is growing epidemiological evidence that long-term use of folate supplements reduces risk (Giovannucci *et al.*, 1998). This is one situation in which nutritional supplementation seems to provide a clear benefit that might be difficult to achieve with diet alone. Clearly, interest in the preventive role of folate-supplemented foods will continue.

Phenolic compounds

A huge variety of biologically active phenolic compounds containing one or more aromatic rings are found naturally in plant foods, where they provide much of the flavour, colour and texture. When tea and alcoholic drinks are taken into account, the daily intake of phenolic substances may be as high as 1 gm per day, even in industrialised societies, but the daily intake of biologically active flavonoids probably amounts to no more than a few tens of mg per day. Flavonoids are very effective antioxidants, although their effects on the overall antioxidant capacity of the plasma are not clear. Many flavonoids also induce Phase II enzymes, suppress the production of biologically active prostaglandins by inhibiting the arachidonic acid cascade, and inhibit mitosis by inhibiting intracellular protein kinases (Formica & Regelson, 1995).

Another large group of phenolic compounds derived from plant foods are classed as phytoestrogens because of their strong similarity to mammalian estrogens (Setchell & Cassidy, 1999). The glycosides genistin and daidzin, and their methylated derivatives biochanin A and formononetin, which are found principally in soya products, are broken down by the intestinal microflora to yield genistein, daidzein, and in some individuals, equol. These products are absorbed into the circulation and their breakdown products can be detected in human urine. The lignan precursors matairesinol and secoisolariciresinol occur more commonly in cereal seeds such as flax, and are degraded in the gut to yield the active lignans enterolactone and enterodiol. In human feeding trials with soya products, isoflavones have been shown to modify the menstrual cycle. In principle these compounds could suppress the growth of hormone-dependent tumours of the breast and prostate (Setchell & Cassidy, 1999), but this remains to be established.

Glucosinolate breakdown products

Brassica vegetables such as cabbage, sprouts, kale and broccoli may offer particularly strong protection against cancer of the lung and gastrointestinal tract (Verhoeven *et al.*, 1996). The brassicas are the only source of glucosinolates, a complex group of compounds all of which contain sulphur, a variable side-chain and a glucose group (Mithen *et al.*, 2000). When the plant tissue is damaged, glucosinolates are hydrolysed by myrosinase, releasing glucose and various breakdown products including isothiocyanates. These hot and bitter compounds are the principle source of flavour in mustard, radishes and the brassica vegetables (Mithen *et al.*, 2000).

Isothiocyanates can selectively induce Phase II enzymes, both in experimental models and human subjects, and there is growing evidence that they suppress tumour development by inducing apoptosis (Smith *et al.*, 1998). In an epidemiological study, Lin *et al.* (1998) observed a protective effect of broccoli against adenomatous polyps, but only in subjects lacking a gene for the expression of a particular form of the Phase II enzyme, glutathione-S-transferase (GST). Isothiocyanates are probably conjugated and excreted more slowly in subjects who do not express GST-μ, so that exposure of target tissues would be more prolonged. This study implies that brassicas might be particularly beneficial to a population sub-group, amounting to about 40% of the population in the UK, and highlights the complex effects of genetic polymorphisms on health.

Conclusions

There is growing evidence that diet acts primarily at the post-initiation stages of human cancer, largely through the provision of protective factors. There is growing evidence that so-called phytoprotectants are at least as important in this regard as the micronutrients as we conventionally define them. The mechanisms of action of both groups of compounds are complex, but our growing understanding of dietary anticarcinogens is likely to lead to much more effective strategies for cancer prevention in the future. These may eventually blur the boundaries between nutrition and pharmacology. In the meantime the epidemiological evidence amply justifies a high and varied consumption of plant foods, with particular emphasis on fruits and vegetables.

References

Albanes, D., Heinonen, O.P., Huttunen, J.K., Taylor, P.R., Virtamo, J., Edwards, B.K., Haapakoski, J., Rautalathi, M., Hartman, A.M., Palmgren, J. & Greenwald, P. (1995) Effects of alpha-tocopherol and beta carotene supplements on cancer incidence I the alpha-tocopherol beta-carotene cancer prevention study. *Am. J. Clin. Nutr.*, **62**, 1427S-30S.

Block, G., Patterson, B. & Subar, A. (1992) Fruit, vegetables, and cancer prevention: a review of the epidemiological evidence. *Nutr. Cancer*, **18**, 1-29.

Bodmer, W.F. (1994) Cancer genetics. *Br. Med. Bull.*, **50**, 517-26.

Doll, R. & Peto, R. (1981) The causes of cancer: quantitative estimates of avoidable risk in the United States. *JNCI*, **66**, 1191-308.

Formica, J.V. & Regelson, W. (1995) Review of the biology of quercetin and related bioflavonoids. *Food. Chem. Toxicol.*, **33**, 1061-80.

Giovannucci, E. Stampfer, M.J., Colditz, G.A., Hunter, D.J., Fuchs, C., Rosner, B.A., Speizer, F.E. & Willett, W.C. (1998) Multivitamin use, folate, and colon cancer in women in the Nurses' Health Study. *Ann. Intern. Med.*, **129**, 517-24.

Greenberg, E.R,. Baron, J.A., Tosteson, T.D., Freeman, D.H., Jr., Beck, G.J., Bond, J.H., Colacchio, T.A., Coller, J.A., Frankl, H.D. & Haile, R.W. (1994) A clinical trial of antioxidant vitamins to prevent colorectal adenoma. Polyp Prevention Study Group. *N. Engl. J. Med.*, **331**, 141-7.

Halliwell, B. (1994) Free radicals and antioxidants: a personal view. *Nutr. Rev.*, **52**, 253-65.

Johnson, I., Williamson, G. & Musk, S. (1994) Anticarcinogenic factors in plant foods: a new class of nutrients? *Nutr. Res. Rev.*, **7**.

Khachik, F., Beecher, G.R. & Smith, J.C. Jr. (1995) Lutein, lycopene, and their oxidative metabolites in chemoprevention of cancer. *J. Cell. Biochem. Suppl.*, **22**, 236-46.

Lin, H.J. Probst-Hensch, N.M., Louie, A.D., Kau, I.H., Witte, J.S., Ingles, S.A.,

Frankl, H.D., Lee, E.R. & Haile, R.W. (1998) Glutathione transferase null genotype, broccoli, and lower prevalence of colorectal adenomas. *Cancer Epidemiol. Biomarkers Prev.*, **7**, 647-52.

Lutz, W.K. & Schlatter, J. (1992) Chemical carcinogens and overnutrition in diet-related cancer. *Carcinogenesis*, **13**, 2211-16.

Ma, J. Stampfer, M.J., Giovannucci, E., Artigas, C.. Hunter, D.J., Fuchs, C., Willett, W.C., Selhub, J., Hennekens, C.H. & Rozen, R. (1997) Methylenetetrahydrofolate reductase polymorphism, dietary interactions, and risk of colorectal cancer. *Cancer Res.*, **57**, 1098-102.

Mithen, R.F., Dekker, M., Verkerk, R., Rabot, S. & Johnson, I.T. (2000) The nutritional significance, biosynthesis and bioavailability of glucosinolates in human foods. *J. Sci. Food Agric.*, **80**, 967-84.

Setchell, K.D. & Cassidy, A. (1999) Dietary isoflavones: biological effects and relevance to human health. *J. Nutr.*, **129**, 758S-67S.

Smith, T.K., Lund, E.K., Johnson, I.T. (1998) Inhibition of dimethylhydrazine-induced aberrant crypt foci and induction of apoptosis in rat colon following oral administration of the glucosinolate sinigrin. *Carcinogenesis*, **19**, 267-73.

Tanchou, S. (1843) Recherches sur la frequence du cancer. *Gazette des hopiteaux*, July.

Verhoeven, D.T., Goldbohm, R.A., van Poppel, G., Verhagen, H. & van den Brandt, P.A. (1996) Epidemiological studies on brassica vegetables and cancer risk. *Cancer Epidemiol. Biomarkers Prev.*, **5**, 733-48.

Wattenburg, L. (1990) Inhibition of carcinogenesis by minor anutrient constituents of the diet. *Proc. Nutr. Soc.*, 173-83.

World Cancer Research Fund (1997) *Food, Nutrition and the Prevention of Cancer: A World Perspective*, pp. 216-51. American Institute for Cancer Research, Washington DC.

14

DIETARY INTERVENTION STUDIES AND CANCER PREVENTION

PIETER VAN'T VEER

Introduction

Based on results from observational epidemiological research, it has been estimated that about one third of all cancers in Western societies are attributable to dietary factors. Studies on biological mechanisms have suggested that a large variety of bioactive compounds may interfere with the process of carcinogenesis. To understand the relation between diet intervention studies and cancer prevention, we need to recognise the dimensions of both diet and carcinogenesis. Then, trials can be characterised in terms of these two dimensions, which also indicates their strengths and limitations. This approach will clarify the role of dietary studies in cancer prevention and help us to avoid misinterpretation of the scientific evidence on diet and cancer.

Dimensions of diet and cancer

Diet can be characterised in terms of food pattern (e.g., vegetarian, omnivorous, mediterranean), food groups (e.g., vegetables, fruits, cereals, meat (products), fats and oils), macronutrients (e.g., fats, animal protein), micronutrients (e.g., vitamins A, C, E, calcium, selenium), phytochemicals (e.g. quercetin, lignans) etc. Regarding cancer, the multistage process of carcinogenesis, lasting decades, is of crucial importance in understanding both the role of diet and the difficulties of 'proving' this association by means of intervention trials. Cancer can be studied at the level of epidemiology (e.g. incidence or mortality of cancer or its clinical precursor lesions), at the clinical level (e.g. precursor lesions like adenomatous polyps or tissue proliferation) or at the biological level (e.g. altered gene expression by mutation or methylation and genetic susceptibility by familial syndromes or polymorphic genes). In our research programme at the Division of Human Nutrition at Wageningen University, we usually label these levels as 'population', 'individual' and 'cell'.

Micronutrient intervention trials and cancer prevention

The Finnish alpha-tocopherol beta-carotene (ATBC) lung cancer trial is the prototype of cancer prevention studies (ATBC, 1994). This was a two-by-two factorial designed randomised, placebo-controlled, double-blinded trial. The study was conducted among a high-risk group for lung cancer, i.e. 57 year old males, who smoked 20 cigarettes per day for an average duration of 36 years. During the 7 (range 5–8) years of follow-up four groups of these men (14 600 per group) used supplements with AT (50 mg/day), BC (20 mg/day), either alone or in combination and placebo. After seven years of follow-up neither AT nor BC showed any evidence of protection against lung cancer. Another study on BC, vitamin A and lung cancer showed similar results (Omenn, 1996). Analyses on other cancer endpoints from the ATBC study and from the Linxian intervention study in China suggested that BC and/or AT (Heinonen *et al.*, 1998; Varis *et al.*, 1998; Rautalahti *et al.*, 1999; Albanes *et al.*, 2000) or a combination of vitamins and minerals is not likely to reduce cancer risk (Blot *et al.*, 1993). Possible exceptions are AT in prostate cancer (ATBC), a combination of BC, AT and selenium (Se) in stomach cancer (Linxian) and Se in the prevention of second primaries among subjects who earlier had skin cancer (Clarck *et al.*, 1997) (Figure 14.1). The strengths of these types of studies include that they directly address the clinically relevant endpoint, that the dietary component is well-defined and that the design resembles that of randomised controlled clinical trials as used in evaluation of treatment efficacy in drug development. Limitations are that the duration of such trials is limited as compared to the multistage nature of carcinogenesis and that the intervention measures apply to a rather late stage in this process. Furthermore, the dose of supplements usually exceeds the level of dietary intake (not so much in Linxian trial), and that means the components tested cannot be directly generalised to food patterns and dietary advice, e.g. because of their bioavailability. Nevertheless, the largely negative findings of these trials have strengthened the idea from observational epidemiology that dietary sources of BC (e.g. vegetables and fruits) may contain relatively low doses of natural components relevant to cancer prevention.

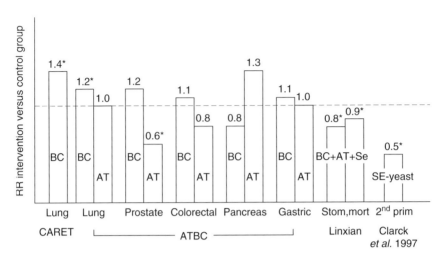

Figure 14.1   Relative risk (RR) of cancer at specific cancer sites after intervention with micronutrients (AT, alpha-tocopherol; BC, beta-carotene; Se, selenium) from CARET, ATBC, Linxian and Clarck *et al.*'s trial (references in text).
*Indicates statistical significant difference from null hypothesis (stom, stomach cancer; mort, total mortality; 2nd prim, second primaries after initial skin cancer).

Micronutrient intervention trials to prevent cancer precursors

One of the first trials in this category was the Australian Polyp Prevention Trial. Instead of clinical cancer, the endpoint of this study was the occurrence of adenomatous polyps in the 4 years after the index colonoscopy (first year of follow-up was excluded from the analyses). Again, this was a randomised, placebo-controlled, double-blind two-by-two factorial trial (Greenberg *et al.*, 1994). It included 864 subjects (190 per arm), at high risk of adenoma occurrence since 55% of them had one prior adenoma removed. Of these subjects, 80% were male, 45% less then 60 years of age. These subjects received BC (25 mg/day), vitamin C plus AT (1000 and 400 mg/day respectively), their combination or placebo. In the second through fourth years 37% developed an adenoma. The relative risk (RR) for BC was 1.01 (0.85–1.20) and it was 1.08 (0.91–1.29) for Vitamin C plus AT. Another adenoma recurrence trial also failed to find a protective effect of BC (MacLennan *et al.*, 1995) as did the Linxian oesophageal dysplasia study for vitamin and mineral supplements (Li *et al.*, 1993) and the US study on selenium (from yeast) and skin cancer recurrence (Clarck *et al.*, 1997). Regarding calcium supplements, however, two studies have suggested a beneficial role of calcium in adenoma recurrence (Baron *et al.*, 1999; Bonithon-Kopp *et al.*, 2000) (Figure 14.2). The strength of these

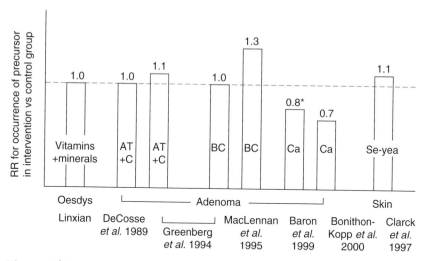

Figure 14.2 Relative risk (RR) for occurrence of precursor lesions of cancer after intervention with micronutrients (AT, alpha-tocopherol; BC, beta-carotene; C, vitamin C; Ca, calcium; Se, selenium) from various trials (references in text; note: Linxian trial addresses cancer mortality among subjects with oesophageal dysplasia).
*Indicates statistical significant difference from null hypothesis.

studies is similar to the previous type of cancer-endpoint trials (RCT-like, components well-defined) as are their limitations (dose, implications for prevention). Furthermore, the high risk groups enrolled in these trials may not fully represent the aetiology in the population at large (because of genetic and/or acquired susceptibility); moreover, the implications of their results highly depend on whether the precursor lesion is indeed part of the causal chain leading to malignancy. Nevertheless, the largely negative results of these trials (with the possible exception of calcium) have diminished the evidence for a role of antioxidants in (colorectal) carcinogenesis. Like the cancer-endpoint studies, they tended to shift the scientific attention to the role of vegetables and fruits or the food pattern as such.

Food intervention trials to prevent cancer precursors

The year 2000 seems to be the year in which results from intervention trials with foods and food patterns (rather than supplements) become available. The endpoint for the three trials published was adenoma recurrence, e.g. the US Polyp Prevention Trial (Schatzkin *et al.*, 2000). This trial contained two parallel groups (about 1000 subjects each) of subjects who had at least one polyp removed in the preceding six months. They were males and females over 35 years of age and they were randomised to either maintain their usual diet or to dietary counselling and support to reduce fat intake to 20% of energy, and to increase the intake of fruits and vegetables and dietary fibre to 3.5 servings per 1000 kcal and 18 g/day, respectively. Data analysis of years 2 through 4 showed no difference in recurrence of adenomas, nor in their adenoma size. The other studies focused on the fibre components in diet but failed to provide any evidence for a protective effect of wheat bran fibre from breakfast cereals and bars (Alberts *et al.*, 2000) or from isphagula husk (Bonithon-Kopp *et al.*, 2000) (Figure 14.3). The strength of these studies is that they do not need to identify specific components to be studied, but that they address adaptations of the food pattern within a feasible range which may be directly applicable to the general population. Therefore, their results might be closely related to those obtained from observational studies on precursor lesions. Unfortunately, their limitations are similar to those of the former category of trials. Moreover, the limitations also resemble those from observational epidemiology (no double blinding, confounding, i.e. no specific components can be identified). Nevertheless, it seems clear that the food pattern (or foods) evaluated do not directly affect risk of adenoma recurrence in these subjects.

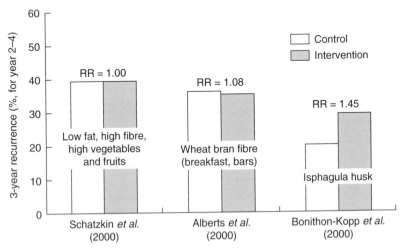

Figure 14.3   Crude three-year cumulative incidence (CI) of adenomatous polyps after intervention with different foods. The adjusted relative risks (RRs) compare the CIs in the intervention versus the control group; RR for the third study was estimated from the odds ratio presented by the authors.

Molecular epidemiology

The former paragraphs suggest (by the method of elimination) that earlier stages of carcinogenesis need to be studied and that the precise relation between adenomas and carcinomas requires scientific attention. Based on evidence from observational epidemiology and laboratory model systems (*in vitro, in vivo*) and on developments in molecular analytical methodology, it now becomes possible to study these stages of carcinogenesis in epidemiological studies. We recently obtained two grants from the Netherlands Organisation for Scientific Research in this newly emerging field of molecular epidemiology.

The first study addresses early stages in colorectal carcinogenesis. This is a two-by-two factorial designed intervention study among subjects who had an adenoma removed at colonoscopy. The intervention in this randomised placebo-controlled double-blinded study is with folate plus vitamin B_{12} and the second factor is the MTHFR genotype (either TT or CC). Results will include vitamin concentrations in blood and recto-sigmoidal biopsies, DNA-methylation and synthesis in the biopsies. In addition, differential gene analysis will be conducted using micro-array technology, both under controlled *in vitro* cellular models as in the biopsies. The second study addresses the later stages in colorectal carcinogenesis. It includes a collaboration between the Wageningen adenoma case control study and the Netherlands Cohorts Study on diet and cancer (NLCS) by Maastricht University and the TNO Institutes. These studies already included vegetables, fruits and meat products as dietary factors. The present grant aims to extend this with mutation patterns (in APC, beta-catenin and K-ras) and polymorphisms in GST and NAT coding regions, both in adenomas and carcinomas.

The total of about 600 adenoma cases and 800 carcinoma cases allows us to study both dietary factors (food and nutrient intake) and genetic susceptibility (polymorphisms) in relation to specific endpoints (mutations) at different stages of colorectal carcinogenesis (adenomas, carcinomas). These molecular epidemiological studies may help to develop a coherent interpretation of the available evidence from both intervention studies and observational epidemiology. This will help to further substantiate dietary guidelines advice as a basis for cancer prevention.

Future research

The rapidly growing field of molecular research opens new approaches for research aiming at cancer prevention. Using laboratory technologies it becomes possible to zoom in on relevant categories of components by screening a wide spectrum of mixtures and components using a large range of cellular and animal models with different sensitivity to these compounds. Both dosing of exposure and time to effect can be studied in these models, which is relevant to causal interpretation of human intervention and observational studies. Of course, limitations include that these approaches rely heavily on cellular and animal models. Thus, digestion, absorption, distribution, metabolism and excretion in humans is 'bypassed', and results need to be verified in human studies. Thus, as illustrated in the former paragraph, based on insight into the process of carcinogenesis, molecular-based types of intervention studies and observational studies are likely to appear in the near future.

Strategies towards cancer prevention

How can current scientific evidence be translated into strategies for cancer prevention at the population level?

First, by improving food safety, aiming to avoid exposure to (pre)carcinogens, that is by excluding (geno)toxicity, e.g. by proper methods of food storage (prevention of aflatoxins) and food preparation habits (barbecuing, meat preparation).

Second, by improving food patterns, i.e. by public education to optimise habitual food choice and dietary habits regarding consumption of vegetables and fruits, limiting alcohol consumption and control of body weight.

Third, the role of industry might gradually increase because ongoing research may lead to efficacious functional foods, allowing substantiated functional claims and even health claims.

Fourth, research among high risk groups (risk families, polypectomised subjects) may lead to advising specific supplements. As illustrated, this approach has not been successful so far. Moreover, the use of supplements should primarily be viewed as a research method and pharmacological approach, rather than a public health strategy.

Finally, some groups advocate the use micronutrients in high doses far beyond the nutritional range. Again, this is mainly of pharmacological and toxicological interest. However, its application to human cancer prevention is based on a misunderstanding of scientific evidence and/or principles.

Conclusion

The contribution of intervention studies to cancer prevention can be summarised as follows. Regarding food patterns and macronutrients, intervention trials will help to strengthen evidence on mechanisms by which diet may affect carcinogenesis. These are likely to be too expensive and will lack the methodological strength required to obtain validly quantitative estimates of cancer risk. Regarding micronutrients and phytochemicals, intervention trials may help bridge the gap between observational epidemiology and laboratory research and some of them may even be able to quantify the strength of such an association, either for cancer precursors or for cancer incidence.

Nevertheless, the interpretation of intervention studies will always be hindered by the multistage nature of cancer, which limits the usefulness of studying a selected number of components over a relatively limited period of time. In order to connect the pieces of evidence from the different lines of research, the growing attention for molecular epidemiological and laboratory research needs to be paralleled by mathematical and statistical modelling of the diet: cancer association. In conclusion, dietary guidelines for cancer prevention are public health measures, they are based on the best estimates derived from the evidence currently available, and therefore they are subject to change and refinement when newer and stronger evidence emerges.

References

Albanes, D., Malila, N., Taylor, P.R. *et al.* (2000) Effects of supplemental alpha-tocopherol and beta-carotene on colorectal cancer: results from a controlled trial (Finland). *Cancer Causes Control*, **11**, 197–205.

Alberts, D.S., Martinez, M.E., Roe, D.J. *et al.* (2000) Lack of effect of a high-fiber cereal supplement on the recurrence of colorectal adenomas. *New. Eng. J. Med.*, **342**, 1156–62.

ATBC (1994) Alpha-tocopherol, beta-carotene cancer prevention study group. The effect of vitamin E and beta-carotene on the incidence of lung cancer and other cancers in male smokers. *New Eng. J. Med.*, **330**, 1029–35.

Baron, J.A., Beach, M., Mandel, J.S. *et al.* (1999) Calcium supplements for the prevention of colorectal adenomas. *N. Eng. J. Med.*, **340**, 101–7.

Blot, W.J., Li, J.Y., Taylor, P.R. *et al.* (1993) Nutrition intervention trials in Linxian, China: supplementation with specific vitamin/mineral combinations, cancer incidence, and disease-specific mortality in the general population. *J. Natl. Cancer Inst.*, **85**, 1483–92.

Bonithon-Kopp, C., Kronborg, O., Giacosa, A. *et al.* (2000) Calcium and fibre supplementation in prevention of colorectal adenoma recurrence: a randomised intervention trial. *Lancet*, **356**, 1300–1306.

Clarck, L.C., Combs, G.F., Turnbull, B.W. *et al.* (1997) Effects of selenium supplementation for cancer prevention in patients with carcinoma of the skin. *J. Am. Med. Assoc.*, **276**, 1957–63.

DeCosse, J.J., Miller, H.H. & Lesser, M.L. (1989) Effect of wheat fiber and vitamins C and E on rectal polyps in patients with familial adenomatous polyposis. *J. Natl. Cancer Inst.*, **81**, 1290–97.

Greenberg, E.R., Baron, J.A., Tosteson, T.D. *et al.* (1994) A clinical trial of antioxidant vitamins to prevent colorectal adenoma. *N. Eng. J. Med.*, **331**, 141–7.

Heinonen, P.O., Albanes, D., Virtamo, J. *et al.* (1998) Prostate cancer and supplementation with alpha-tocopherol and beta-carotene: incidence and mortality in a controlled trial. *J. Natl. Cancer Inst.*, **90**, 440–46.

Li, J.Y., Taylor, P.R., Lui, B. *et al.* (1993) Nutrition intervention trials in Linxian, China: multiple vtiamin/mineral supplementation, cancer incidence, and disease-specific mortality among adults with oesophageal dysplasia. *J. Natl. Cancer Inst.*, **85**, 1492–8.

MacLennan, R., Macrae, F., Bain, C. *et al.* (1995) Randomized trial of intake of fat, fiber, and beta-carotene to prevent colorectal adenomas. *J. Natl. Cancer Inst.*, **87**, 1760–66.

Omenn, G.S., Goodman, G.E., Thornquist, M.D. *et al.* (1996) Risk factors for lung cancer and for intervention effects in CARET, the beta-carotene and retinol efficacy trial. *J. Natl. Cancer Inst.*, **88**, 1550–59.

Rautalahti, M.T., Virtamo, J.R.K., Taylor, P.R. *et al.* (1999) The effects of supplementation with alpha-tocopherol and beta-carotene on the incidence and mortality of carcinoma of the pancreas in a randomized, controlled trial. *Cancer*, **86**, 37–42.

Schatzkin, A., Lanza, E., Corle, D. *et al.* (2000) Lack of effect of a low-fat, high-fiber diet on the recurrence of colorectal adenomas. *New Eng. J. Med.*, **342**, 1149–55.

Varis, K., Taylor, P.R., Sipponen, P. *et al.* (1998) Gastric cancer and premalignant lesions in atrophic gastritis: a controlled trial on the effect of supplementation with alpha-tocopherol and beta-carotene. *Scand. J. Gastroenterol.*, **33**, 294–300.

15

DIABETES:
FAMILIAL, GENETIC OR LIFESTYLE?

ANNE DORNHORST

Introduction

We are currently experiencing a pan-epidemic of type 2 diabetes in the developed world. Between 1958 and 1994 there was a five-fold increase in the prevalence of type 2 diabetes in the USA. Similar increases have occurred in the UK, where today's prevalence for type 2 diabetes is around 2–4% for the adult population, with higher prevalence rates occurring among the Indian Asians and Afro-Caribbean populations. This rise in type 2 diabetes is due to an already present underlying genetic susceptibility to type 2 diabetes becoming expressed under the influences of today's lifestyle that promotes weight gain and physical inactivity. These lifestyle changes are compounded by the additional influences of the maternal transmission of diabetes to children born to mothers with diabetes; this effect is independent of any genetic influence and attributable to fetal exposure to hyperglycaemia in utero. As type 2 diabetes is now firmly established among women of child bearing age the importance of maternal transmission of diabetes is increasing.

Genetic susceptibility of type 2 diabetes

There is without doubt a strong genetic susceptibility to type 2 diabetes. It has been recognised for many years that type 2 diabetes aggregates within families and among certain ethnic groups. While 10–30% of first degree relatives of type 2 diabetic subjects are themselves diabetic, this drops to 1–6% among first degree relatives of non-diabetic subjects. The importance of genetic factors is further illustrated by a greater than 70% concordance rate for type 2 diabetes among monozygotic twins compared with less than 30% among dizygotic twins.

While genetic factors are clearly important in determining an individual's potential risk for developing type 2 diabetes, an interaction between this genetic susceptibility and environmental factors is often required before the disease actually manifests. The interaction between a dormant genetic susceptibility to type 2 diabetes and permissive environmental factors is highlighted by studies on populations that migrate from areas with a low prevalence of diabetes to areas with a high prevalence rate. Type 2 diabetes is rare in rural India; however when individuals migrate to the West the prevalence of type 2 diabetes rises sharply.

Type 2 diabetes is usually a polygenic disorder; it is generally believed that a number of key genes influence different aspects of carbohydrate and fat metabolism, which together contribute to the genetic risk of type 2 diabetes. There are however a number of rare monogenic conditions, over 70 in all, that together account for approximately 2% of all known diabetes.

Environmental factors

The current pan-epidemic of type 2 diabetes cannot be explained by genetic factors alone, as the increase in its prevalence rate has occurred faster than any change in the genetic make-up of the population could possibly have taken place. To find the reasons for the rise in type 2 diabetes one needs to look no further than today's lifestyle patterns. Since World War II the rates of obesity in the West have paralleled the rates of type 2 diabetes and this has occurred alongside a dramatic increase in fat consumption and decrease in physical activity. These three lifestyle changes have all independently been shown in large prospective epidemiological studies to be associated with an increased risk for type 2 diabetes. Metabolic studies complement these epidemiological studies by showing that increasing weight and dietary fat consumption as well as decreased physical activity all independently increase insulin resistance. One of the most important metabolic contributors to the development of type 2 diabetes is increased insulin resistance.

Lessons from the Pima Indians

The Pima Indians from Arizona have the highest prevalence of obesity and type 2 diabetes in the world. One half of all adult Pima Indians in Arizona have type 2 diabetes and 95% of these individuals are overweight. The

Pima Indians in Arizona are believed to have originated from descendants of the Hohokam, a prehistoric group of Paleoindians who originally migrated across the Bering Land Bridge from Asia to Mexico and who around 300 BC moved from Mexico to the Gila River valley in Arizona. Over the last 1000 years, Native Americans from north-west Mexico have continued to migrate to the Gila River valley.

Today, there is a cognate branch of the Pima Indians from Arizona who still live in the Sierra Madre Mountains, a remote undeveloped area of north-west Mexico. The Mexican Pima Indians have significantly less obesity and type 2 diabetes than found in Arizona. The prevalence of diabetes in those living in the Sierra Madre Mountains is <6.4% compared with 54% in the those Pima Indians living in Arizona. The Mexican Pima Indians derive a subsistence existence from toiling the land, consuming a traditional diet comprising 13% protein, 23% fat, 63% CHO, <1% alcohol, >50% fibre. The adults in this community spend over 40 hours a week in hard physical labour. All this is in stark contrast to their genetically related cousins from Arizona, whose diet contains >40% fat, with hard physical labour accounting for less than 10 hours per week.

Diabetes was in fact extremely rare among the Pima Indians in Arizona until the twentieth century; Dr Joslin from the Boston Clinic actually commented on its low prevalence in an article of the time. The reason for this was that Pima Indians in Arizona maintained their traditional lifestyle up until 1900; at this time they were successful farmers having developed and introduced land irrigation to their crops. However at the beginning of the last century their water supply was diverted by white farmers and they suddenly become dependent on the US government for food which was provided in the form of lard, sugar and white flour. Over the last century the Pima Indians from Arizona have moved into reservations, becoming even more dependent on processed high calorie foods provided for them by the US Government. Hard physical work in the field is now only a distant memory.

It is now believed that the Pima Indians whether from Arizona or the Mexican Sierra Madre Mountains have a strong genetic predisposition to type 2 diabetes that affects up to 50% of the population. However manifestation of this genetic predisposition requires interaction from environmental factors. An interesting explanation of how susceptible the Pima Indians are to type 2 diabetes is that the genes for type 2 diabetes are the very genes that protected their ancestors over many generations from malnutrition and intermittent famines – the so-called 'thrifty gene theory'.

The thrifty gene theory

Professor Neel (1962) suggested that populations whose survival relied on food from the land and who were likely to experience alternating periods of feast and famine, developed by natural selection a thrifty gene that facilitated fat deposition during times of plenty to protect against times of famine. This hypothesis is illustrated well by the metabolic phenotype of the Pima Indians who are characterised as having insulin resistance and central obesity, both traits known to be strongly genetically determined. Insulin resistance is beneficial during times of food shortage as it helps divert glucose away from skeletal muscle to the brain; and at times of food surplus insulin resistance maximises fat disposition. Another survival benefit of insulin resistance is during pregnancy: this facilitates the maternal-fetal transfer of fuels substrates, protecting the fetus nutritionally at the expense of the mother. Although a degree of maternal insulin resistance is advantageous during pregnancy, maternal diabetes is not. An important consequence of the recent rise in type 2 diabetes is the adverse influence that maternal diabetes is having on programming fetal metabolism, which is further fuelling the current epidemic of type 2 diabetes.

Type 2 diabetes and the intrauterine environment

The literature supports a stronger maternal than paternal transmission of type 2 diabetes. Children born to diabetic mothers have a greater risk of both obesity and type 2 diabetes than their older siblings, born to the same mother at a time when she was not diabetic. Maternal diabetes accounts for 40% of all type 2 diabetes in Pima Indian children (5–19 years). A two to three-fold increase in the prevalence of type 2 diabetes has been documented in both Pima Indian girls and boys over the last 30 years. In this population over 70% of subjects exposed to maternal diabetes are themselves diabetic at 25–34 years. Diabetes in the mother brings out diabetes in the children at an earlier age than occurs when the mother is not diabetic. In addition, offspring of mothers with diabetes in pregnancy have a much higher prevalence of severe obesity in early adolescence. It has become increasingly recognised that maternal metabolic programming of fetal metabolism occurs, and this is relevant to the development of diabetes and obesity in post-natal life. More recently early neonatal feeding has also been shown to be a possible influence on the future risk of type 2 diabetes. Pettitt *et al.* (1997) showed that among a cohort of 741 Pima Indians children followed for 29 years, those that were exclusively breastfed developed less type 2 diabetes by the age of 30–39 years than those who were exclusively bottle-fed, 20% versus 30%.

Solution to the rising epidemic of type 2 diabetes

The human and monetary costs of the current rising epidemic of type 2 diabetes are enormous: approximately 16% of the American and 7% of the UK total health care budget is being spent on the care of diabetes and its complications. It is now clear that lifestyle habits impact on genetic factors to cause type 2 diabetes. The onset of type 2 diabetes is now occurring at a younger age and has become common among women of child bearing age. Maternal diabetes is now another important contributor to obesity and diabetes in young adult life. Public health measures in terms of healthy living advice are urgently required to stem today's current pan-epidemic in type 2 diabetes.

References

Neel, Professor (1962) Diabetes mellitus: a thrithy genotype rendered detrimental by 'progress'. *Am. J. Hum. Gen.*, **14**, 353–362.

Petitt, D.J., Forman, M.R., Hanson, R.L., Knowler, W.C. & Bennett P.H. (1997) Breastfeeding and the incidence of non-insulin-dependent diabetes mellitus in Pima Indians. *Lancet*, **350**, 166–8.

Suggested reading

Dabelea, D., Knowler, W.C. & Pettitt, D. (2000) The effect of diabetes in pregnancy on offspring: follow-up research in the Pima Indians. *J. Meterna-Fetal. Med.*, **9**, 83–8.

Kriska, A.M., LaPorte, R.E., Pettitt, D.J., Charles, M.A., Nelson, R.G., Kuller, L.H., Bennett, P.H. & Knowler, W.C. (1993) The association of physical activity with obesity, fat distribution and glucose intolerance in Pima Indians. *Diabetologia*, **36**, 863–9.

Ravussin, E., Valencia, M.E., Esparza, J., Bennett, P.H. & Schulz, L.O. (1999) Effects of a traditional lifestyle on obsesity in Pima Indians. *Diabetes Care*, **17**, 1067–74.

Sakul, H., Pratley, R., Cardon, L., Ravussin, E., Mott, D. & Bogardus, C. (1997) Familiality of physical and metabolic characteristics that predict the development of non-insulin dependent diabetes mellitus in Pima Indians. *Am. J. Hum. Genet.*, **60**, 651–6.

16

DIETARY CONTROL OF DIABETES

GARY FROST

Carbohydrate has always played a role in the management of people with diabetes. In the 1900s, before the advent of insulin therapy, the only method of treating type 1 diabetes was by total restriction of carbohydrate. Carbohydrate restriction played a role through most of the twentieth century; even today people with diabetes are still asked to restrict carbohydrate foods such as grapes without any scientific reason. In the early 1980s, the first set of dietary guidelines for people with diabetes recommended that carbohydrate should form 50% of total energy. This carbohydrate should form a 'complexed' source which was 'unrefined'. This had the effect of turning the nutritional advice for people with diabetes 'brown' due to the encouragement of large amounts of wheat fibre. Today we are still left with this inheritance. The aim of this chapter is to review this.

The messages from research into diabetes to improve quality of life are very simple. Results from the Diabetes Control and Complication Study (DCCT, 2001) and the United Kingdom Prospective Diabetes Study (UKPDS, 1998) are very similar for both type 1 and type 2 diabetes. Glycaemic control is important – the closer it is to normal levels, the less risk of complication. Achieving this usually means a greater risk of hypoglycaemic episodes. The largest cause of mortality in the diabetes population is heart disease. It is important that dietary advice reflects this. As carbohydrate contributes to a large percentage of total energy intake, it is important to know how carbohydrates may influence these outcome measures.

Carbohydrates are a complex group ranging from the very simple molecule such as glucose to the very complex such as amylopectin and hemicellulose. They can have different properties depending on processing; also their susceptibility to enzymes such as amylase varies, independent of chain length. Classifying carbohydrates on chemical analysis alone gives very little impression of their physiological effects. This is what was fundamentally wrong with systems such as carbohydrate exchange systems. A given weight of carbohydrate from two different foods can give major differences in glycaemic response. For example, bread will give a very rapid response whereas pasta gives a slower postprandial response. This would not be taken into account on a traditional system that bases the diet solely on chemical measurement of carbohydrate. This is the basis for glycaemic index.

Dietary fibre

Dietary fibre is a complex group. I will focus here on the effect of fibre on blood glucose and lipid metabolism. As stated above, the first dietary guideline had the effect of increasing the amount of carbohydrate.

The term dietary fibre refers to non-starch polysaccharides and lignin present in plant products. They are a diverse group, and in general are not digested in the upper gastrointestinal tract. There are many ways of classifying dietary fibre from the metabolic view. It is probably best classified as either water-soluble, with the ability to form viscous gels, or insoluble in water (Table 16.1).

Table 16.1   Classification of dietary fibre.

Water soluble	Water insoluble
• Hemicelluloses	• Celluloses
• Pectins	• Resistant starch
• Gums	
• Mucilages	
• Carageenan	
• Agar	

It is the water-soluble fibres which have been reported to have significant positive effects on postprandial glucose concentration and lipid levels. Wheat fibre has very little metabolic effect; encouraging wholemeal bread has little effect on glycaemic control. Foods that have a high soluble fibre such as beans and pulse vegetables have been consistently demonstrated to have positive effects.

Guar gum

There is much literature not only pertaining to guar gum but also many soluble fibre supplements such as sugar beet fibre, pectin and psyllium. It is fair to say that some of the products were doomed to failure and hence this has created a small amount of negative literature. This, coupled with poor gastrointestinal side effects, has condemned products like guar gum to be left out of everyday clinical usage. However, I think there needs to be a new look. Soluble fibres, to have their effects, need to be fully hydrated; a number of products around the early 1980s which were developed to aid diabetes management never fully hydrated. There is also clear evidence to demonstrate that these fibre supplements work best when mixed intimately and hydrated within a food matrix. Evidence suggests that by using defined molecular weight products with a known effect on viscosity, a fraction of the total weight of the supplement is needed in order to have a clinically significant effect on glycaemic control and lipid metabolism. This has the effect of reducing the gastrointestinal side-effects enormously. A very encouraging study by Peter Ellis (Kings College, University of London) and Peter Frost (Central Middlesex Hospital) involved people with type 2 diabetes being given guar-enriched bread over a 6-week period, and the results showed significant improvement in glycaemic control and lipid levels (unpublished data).

The mechanism of action is possibly a mixture of the following:

• Slowing of gastric emptying
• Effects on glucose diffusion towards the brush border of the intestine
• Changes in the unstirred layer
• Effects on rates of enzyme digestion
• Effects on release of gut peptides
• Effects on starch granules

I feel these positive results cannot be ignored.

Glycaemic index

It has been known for many years that different carbohydrate foods with the same macronutrient composition produce different glycaemic responses. The systematic classification of carbohydrate foods according to their glycaemic response was first done by Otto *et al* (1973). The idea was to keep the glycaemic impact of the diet the same regardless of the variety of carbohydrate used. The same author described differences not only in glucose but also insulin response. Jenkins *et al.* (1981) coined the term glycaemic index in the early 1980s and since then it has been a major topic of discussion over its applicability to the management of diabetes mellitus. Recently some important landmarks show that the glycaemic index deserves a place in clinical practice:

(1) The WHO/FAO report suggestion that the physiological effects of carbohydrate should be classified by glycaemic index (FAO/WHO, 1998).
(2) Evidence suggesting that people who habitually consume a diet rich in slowly absorbed carbohydrate (low glycaemic index) have reduced risk of type 2 diabetes and coronary heart disease (Salmeron *et al.*, 1997; Frost *et al.*, 1999).
(3) A strengthening of the evidence of the usefulness of glycaemic index in the clinical management of diabetes mellitus.
(4) The link between high glycaemic index diets with insulin resistance and type 2 diabetes and cardiovascular disease (CVD) (Dornhorst & Frost, 2000).

Therefore I conclude by advocating that nutritional guidelines for diabetes should place greater emphasis on the glycaemic index.

Definition

The glycaemic indexes of several foods are published in international nutritional tables. Methodology on their derivation is available from previous reviews (Wolever, 1990). In summary, the glycaemic index is a measure of a carbohydrate's post-prandial glucose response. The glycaemic index provides a standardised comparison of a carbohydrate's 2-hour post-prandial glucose response with that of white bread or glucose.

The glycaemic index model

$$\frac{\text{Incremental area under blood glucose response curve for the test food containing 50 g of carbohydrate}}{\text{corresponding area after equi-carbohydrate portion of white bread}} \times 100$$

Low glycaemic index carbohydrates have lower 2-hour areas under the glucose curve than white bread, while high glycaemic index foods have higher areas. Although the insulin response is not part of the glycaemic index calculation, the lower the glycaemic index of a food the more attenuated is the insulin response (Wolever, 1990).

Type of dietary carbohydrate and the glycaemic index

The present classification of carbohydrates is based on chemical analysis of carbohydrate content rather than physiology. The glycaemic index of a carbohydrate, however, is determined more by physiology, being highly dependent on a carbohydrate's absorption rate. The glycaemic index is influenced by a carbohydrate's composition, tertiary structure and enzymic digestion as listed below:

- Amylose and amylopectin ratio
- Relationship of insoluble and soluble non-starch polysaccharides to glycaemic index
- Cell structure
- Food preparation and processing.

The benefits of low glycaemic index carbohydrates on diabetic control

Three month clinical studies have shown that low glycaemic index carbohydrates improve glycaemic control in both type 1 and type 2 diabetes and reduce post-prandial glucose and plasma insulin concentrations in type 2 diabetes (Frost *et al.*, 1994) and post-prandial glucose in type 1 (Wolever *et al.*, 1990). Good glycaemic control and favourable lipid and fibrinolytic profiles have also been reported in individuals with type 1 and type 2 diabetes who habitually consume low glycaemic index dietary carbohydrates (Lafrance *et al.*, 1998). It remains to be shown whether these diets bestow long-term benefits on micro or macro-vascular complications.

The benefits of low glycaemic index carbohydrates on CVD risk factors

High glycaemic index foods induce post-prandial hyperinsulinaemia which is a powerful predictor for metabolic risk factors and CVD in epidemiological studies. Both cross-sectional and prospective population studies have shown favourable lipid profiles in association with low glycaemic index diets. Low glycaemic index diets are associated with reduction in total and LDL-cholesterol, improvement in clotting profiles, and increase in insulin sensitivity. My colleagues and I recently demonstrated an indirect relationship between HDL-cholesterol and glycaemic index. Low glycaemic index diets also lower serum cholesterol and triglyceride levels in hyperlipidaemic subjects.

Conclusions

Carbohydrate is a very complex group of foods. Rather than looking at this group to identify those with a detrimental effect it would be simpler to see some groups of carbohydrates as having a positive effect. The beneficial metabolic effects of soluble fibre and low glycaemic index carbohydrates cannot be ignored. More thought needs to be given to rolling out these concepts into clinical practice. As regards the original aims of diabetes management (i.e. glycaemic control and cardiac risk factor management), both soluble fibre and glycaemic index will help support these.

Acknowledgements.

I am grateful for the help and support of many people including those who work in my own department, as well as Professor Bloom, Dr Leeds and Dr Dornhorst.

References

DCCT (2001) Diabetes Control and Complications Trial Group. The effect of intensive treatement of diabetes on the development and progression of long term complications in insulin dependent diabetes. *N. Eng. J. Med.*, **329**, 977–87.

Dornhorst, A. & Frost, G. (2000) The relevance of the glycaemic index to our understanding of dietary carbohydrates. *Diabet. Med.*, **17**, 336–45.

FAO/WHO (1998) Carbohydrates in human nutrition. *Report of a joint FAO/WHO conference*, Rome 14–18 April 1997. Paper 66. FAO Food and Nutrition.

Frost, G., Leeds, A.R., Dore, C.J., Madeiros, S., Brading, S. & Dornhorst, A. (1999) Glycaemic index as a determinant of serum HDL-cholesterol concentration. *Lancet*, **353**, 1045–8.

Frost, G., Wilding, J. & Beecham, J. (1994) Dietary advice based on the glycaemic index improves dietary profile and metabolic control in type 2 diabetic patients. *Diabet. Med.*, **11**, 397–401.

Jenkins, D.J., Wolever, T.M., Taylor, R.H., Barker, H., Fielden, H., Baldwin, J.M. *et al.* (1981) Glycemic index of foods: a physiological basis for carbohydrate exchange. *Am. J. Clin. Nutr.*, **34**, 362–6.

Lafrance, L., Rabasa-Lhoret, R., Piossin, D., Ducros, F. & Chiassen, J.L. (1998) The effects of different glycaemic index foods and dietary fibre intake on glycaemic control in type 1 diabetic patients on intensive insulin therapy. *Diabet. Med.*, **15**, 972–8.

Otto, H., Bleger, G., Penmartz, M., Subin, G., Scheauberger, G. & Spaethe, K. (1973) Kohlenhydrataustaunch nach biologischen aquivalentnjin. In *Diatetik bei Diabetes Mellitus* (eds H. Otto & R. Spaethe), pp. 41–50. Huber, Bern.

Salmeron, J., Manson, J.E., Stampfer, M.J., Colditz, G.A., Wing, L. L. & Willett, W. (1997) Dietary fiber, glycemic load, and risk of non-insulin-dependent diabetes mellitus in women. *JAMA*, **277** (6), 472–7.

UKPDS (1998) UK Prospective Diabetes Study. Effect of intensive blood-glucose control with metformin on complications in overweight patients with type 2 diabetes (UKPDS 34). *Lancet,* **352** (9131), 854–65.

Wolever, T.M. (1990) The glycemic index. *World Rev. Nutr. Diet.,* **62**, 120–85.

Wolever, T.M., Jenkins, D.J., Collier, G.R., Ehrlich, R.M., Josse, R.G., Wong, G.S. *et al.* (1988) The glycaemic index: effect of age in insulin dependent diabetes mellitus. *Diabetes Res.* **7** (2), 71–4.

17

MANAGEMENT OF THE HUMAN GUT FLORA FOR IMPROVED HEALTH

GLENN R. GIBSON

In the human intestinal tract a huge and diverse range of bacterial species exist, thought to contribute about 95% of all the cells in the body. This microflora plays a significant role in the digestive process and without its activities life would be extremely uncomfortable, if not impossible. In comparison to other regions of the gastrointestinal tract, the human colon is an extremely densely populated microbial ecosystem. Generally, the various components of the large intestinal microbiota may be considered as exerting pathogenic effects or they may have potential health promoting values. For example, certain gut flora components are involved in gastroenteritis and, possibly, more chronic disorders such as ulcerative colitis and bowel cancer. On the other hand, bifidobacteria and lactobacilli are thought to exert protective effects in the gut. Main positive effects associated with their activities have been considered as cholesterol and/or triglyceride reduction, anti-tumour properties, protection against gastroenteritis, improved lactose tolerance and stimulation of the immune system through non-pathogenic means (Gibson & Roberfroid, 1999).

Bacteria in the colon respond largely to the available fermentable substrate, which is mainly provided by foodstuffs unabsorbed or digested by mammalian enzymes. Given that the microbiota have components that may be positive for human health, there is currently much interest in the use of diet to specifically increase groups perceived as health promoting. Two approaches are common.

Probiotics and prebiotics

Probiotics are live microbial feed additions incorporated into the diet. Records of probiotic intake by humans have been taken from as long as over 2000 years ago; however the first scientific evidence of their value was at the start of the 1900s. The founder of probiotics is Ellie Metchnikoff who worked at the Pasteur Institute in Paris (Metchnikoff, 1907). He observed that Bulgarian peasants had longevity and associated this with their elevated intake of 'soured milks' – what we today call probiotics. Over the years many species of microorganisms have been used. They mainly consist of lactic acid producing bacteria (lactobacilli, streptococci, enterococci, lactococci, bifidobacteria) but also *Bacillus* spp. and fungi such as *Saccharomyces* spp. and *Aspergillus* spp. (Fuller, 1992).

A prebiotic is formally defined as 'a non-digestible food ingredient that beneficially affects the host by selectively stimulating the growth and/or activity of one or a limited number of bacteria in the colon, that can improve the host health' (Gibson & Roberfroid, 1995). Thus, the prebiotic approach advocates the administration of non-viable dietary components. At present, most prebiotics are selected on the basis of their ability to promote the growth of lactic acid microorganisms that are already in the gut. Popular prebiotics in current use include oligosaccharides of fructose and galactose as well as lactulose. Other candidate materials include lactosucrose, soybean oligosaccharides, palatinose, isomalto-oligo-saccharides, gluco-oligosaccharides and xylo-oligosaccharides.

Over half the world's population is unable to utilise lactose effectively. The basis for improved digestibility of lactose in probiotics may involve lactase activity of the bacteria or a stimulation of the host's mucosal lactase activity. Various claims have been made for beneficial effects of probiotics and prebiotics against infectious diarrhoea conditions. The manner in which this may occur could be due to the production of strong acids/other antimicrobial compounds, immune stimulation, metabolism of toxins and/or occupation of potential colonisation sites. Bacterial enzymes which convert pre-carcinogens to active carcinogens are produced in the gut but their involvement in the pathogenesis of cancer is unclear. However, some lactic acid bacteria are effective at decreasing the activities of such enzymes. Studies have shown that dietary supplementation can affect plasma cholesterol concentrations and consequently the incidence of coronary heart disease, but the data has been equivocal. Finally, probiotics and prebiotics may stimulate the immune response such that resistance to infectious agents is improved.

A key prerequisite for the successful future of probiotics and prebiotics is to underpin purported health benefits with sound explanations for the mechanism of action. This would exploit well-controlled clinical trials that use up-to-date methodologies such as molecular typing of gut flora changes in response to diet. More directed developments for the future may include the following matters (Gibson *et al.*, 2000).

Increased persistence through the colon

One obvious attribute that an enhanced probiotic or prebiotic would possess is the ability to persist towards distal areas of the colon. Many common diseases of the human large bowel, such as ulcerative colitis and colonic cancer, arise in the left side. As such, enhanced functionality may arise in this part of the colon.

Anti-adhesive properties

An oligosaccharide with prebiotic properties may also have anti-adhesive activities. This would add major functionality to the approach of altering gut pathogenesis. Binding of pathogens to these receptors is the first step in the colonisation process. There is much potential for developing pre-biotics which incorporate such a receptor monosaccharide or oligo-saccharide sequence. These molecules would thereby act as 'decoy' molecules for gut pathogens but would also stimulate benign components of the microbiota. Such multifunctional prebiotics should increase host resistance to infection.

Anti-attenuative properties

The prebiotic concept may be extrapolated further by considering an attenuation of virulence in certain food-borne pathogens. For example, the plant derived carbohydrate cellobiose is able to repress the patho-genicity of *Listeria monocytogenes* through down regulation of its viru-lence factors.

Development of novel prebiotic food ingredients

At the current time, the most widespread use of a prebiotic is inulin which is used as a dietary fibre, bulking agent and fat replacer in several foods. This is, however, a vastly under explored area of research into prebiotics and there is much potential for development of these oligosaccharides into other useful functional ingredients such as sweeteners, surfactants, etc.

Synbiotics

One important development that is finding its way into functional foods is synbiotics. Here, a useful probiotic would be incorporated into an appropriate dietary vehicle with an appropriate prebiotic. The premise is that the selective substrate would be metabolised by the live addition in the gut. This would enhance probiotic survival as well as offer the advantages of both gut microflora management techniques. A synbiotic has been defined as 'a mixture of probiotics and prebiotics that beneficially affects the host by improving the survival and implantation of live microbial dietary supplements in the gastrointestinal tract'. One example is a mixture of probiotic bifidobacteria with prebiotic fructo-oligo-saccharides.

Encapsulation of probiotics with prebiotics

A further approach whereby probiotics could be targeted towards gut delivery would be to protect them through coating procedures. Encapsulation of the probiotic strains should protect them during passage through the stomach and small intestine. This approach could be extended with a view to developing delivery systems that will release probiotic bacteria to the distal colon, a desirable outcome in terms of human health as most large intestinal disorders arise in the left side. Prebiotics which, by definition, enter the large intestine could be used as the encapsulation material.

The future for probiotics and prebiotics rests with realistic identifications of health promoting values and accurate descriptions of how such effects may occur. It may be that certain population groups are more susceptible to the approach of gut flora modulation (e.g. infants, elderly, hospital patients). However, it is likely that the wider approach will be more rational.

References

Fuller, R. (ed.) (1992) *Probiotics: The Scientific Basis*. Chapman & Hall, London.

Gibson, G.R. & Roberfroid, M.B. (1995) Dietary modulation of the human colonic microbiota: introducing the concept of prebiotics. *J. Nutr.*, **125**, 1401–12.

Gibson, G.R. & Roberfroid, M.B. (eds) (1999) *Colonic Microbiota, Nutrition and Health*. Kluwer Academic Publishers, Dordrecht.

Gibson, G.R., Berry Ottaway, P. & Rastall, R.A. (2000) *Prebiotics: New Developments in Functional Foods*. Chandos Publishing Limited, Oxford.

Metchnikoff, E. (1907) *The Prolongation of Life*. William Heinemann, London.

18

DIET AND OSTEOPOROSIS: WHERE ARE WE NOW?

SUSAN A. NEW

Introduction

Predisposition to poor bone health, resulting in osteoporotic fracture, is a major public health problem. It is estimated that 1 in 3 women and 1 in 12 men over the age of 55 years will suffer from osteoporosis, with approximately 90 000 hip fractures occurring last year in the UK alone. Recent estimates suggest an overall cost to the exchequer of £1.8 billion per annum, with each hip fracture costing approximately £20 000, of which 75% (£15 000) is attributable to the residential care and support services in the first and second year after fracture treatment and only £5000 is for the acute surgical cost (Torgerson *et al.*, 2000). Furthermore, the future economic impact of osteoporosis will be phenomenal: by the year 2030 it is considered that elderly people will account for one in four of the adult population, with a projection of the rise in the number of fractures from 1.66 million in 1990 to 6.26 million by 2050 (World Health Organisation, 1994).

There are a number of changes which occur in bone mass with ageing (Figure 18.1). Two mechanisms principally determine adult bone health:

(1) maximum attainment of peak bone mass (PBM) which is achieved during growth and early adulthood
(2) the rate of bone loss with advancing age, with the menopausal years being a time of considerable concern for women.

Both of these aspects are determined by a combination of genetic,

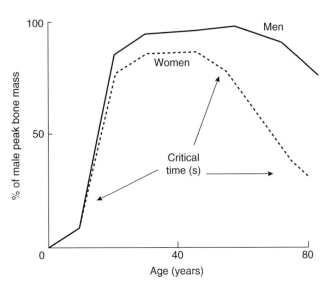

Figure 18.1   Changes in skeletal mass throughout the life cycle. Data from New (2000a).

endocrine, mechanical and nutritional factors, with extensive interactions between them. Studies of bone mass in identical (MZ) and non-identical (DZ) twins and mother: daughter pairs as well as work at the DNA level linking bone mass with a number of gene polymorphisms (including the vitamin D receptor (VDR) gene, oestrogen receptor gene and the collagen type I α 1 gene), suggest that genetic factors account for up to 75% of the variation in bone mass (Ralston, 1999). However, there is still much room for the modifiable factors (such as nutrition and physical activity) to play a vital role in bone health.

Diet and osteoporosis – a review of current knowledge

Role of calcium in peak bone mass attainment and postmenopausal bone loss

Calcium (Ca) is the most abundant mineral element in the body and plays two key roles: structural and regulatory. Bone consists of a protein matrix encased in a crystalline mineral known as hydroxyapatite which contains Ca and phosphate. Approximately 1 kg of Ca is contained within the skeleton (or put another way, 99% of total body Ca is contained within bones and teeth). It is this mineral part of bone which provides its strength as well providing a reserve of Ca which behaves as a large 'ion exchanger',

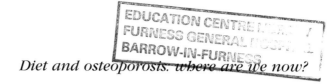
enabling the interaction of Ca ions in body fluid and bone. In its second role, Ca is essential for cellular structure, inter and intracellular metabolic function and signal transmissions and is involved in a number of activities, such as muscle contractions including heart muscle, nerve function, activities of enzymes, and normal clotting of blood. Although only 1% of Ca is found in soft tissues and body fluids, it is this regulatory role that takes precedence over the structural role. Plasma levels are maintained within very narrow limits (90–110 mg/l) by the calciotrophic hormones (Calcitriol (vitamin D), parathyroid hormone (PTH) and calcitonin (CT)) and the Ca contained in the skeleton is sacrificed if the levels of plasma Ca are reduced.

There is considerable controversy as to the importance of calcium (Ca) in PBM development, amongst scientists and clinicians alike both within and between countries. A useful point of note is that the difference in the recommended levels of Ca intake between the UK and the USA may be explained, in part, by the dissimilar way in which they have approached the problem. The UK COMA committee has determined intakes which are deemed adequate for a population whereas the USA NAS panel have targeted intakes that are optimal for health (Weaver, 1999).

Ca supplementation studies in general have shown an association between higher Ca intake and increased bone mineral status (in the order of 1–5%), with the effect greatest in the early stages of supplementation period. However, as shown in Figure 18.2, the strength of this effect is limited due to the findings of some studies that the bone gain disappears

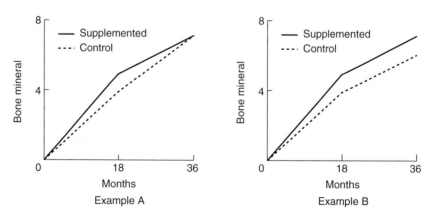

Figure 18.2 Ca supplementation and bone health: short v. long term benefits? Data from New (2000a).

upon withdrawal of the supplement and clearly further research work is required.

As shown in Table 18.1, there is good data to suggest that Ca supplements are effective in reducing bone loss in late menopausal women (>5 years post-menopause), particularly in those with low habitual Ca intake (< 400 mg/d). The study by Dawson-Hughes *et al.* (1990) marked the turning point for studies differentiating between early and late post-menopause. The findings of Ca supplementation studies in the early stages of the menopause are conflicting and this is an area for further investigation (Table 18.2).

Table 18.1 Calcium supplementation studies in peri and early post-menopausal women. Data from New (1999).

Authors	Study duration (yrs)	n	Age (yrs)	TSM[a] (yrs)	Ca-C[b] (mg)	Ca-S[c] (mg)	Ca Effect[d]
Aloia *et al.*, 1994	2.9	101	52	3–6	470	1700	+ve
Elders *et al.*, 1991	3	248	49	1.2	1150	2500	+ve
Dawson-Hughes *et al.*, 1990	2	67	54	< 5	513	1013	No change
Ettinger *et al.*, 1987	2	73	51	< 3	994	2950	No change
Riis *et al.*, 1987	2	36	49	< 3	—	2000	+ve
Nilas *et al.*, 1984	2	103	—	< 3	910	1410	No change

[a] TSM = time since menopause in years; [b] Ca-C = control group calcium intake (mg); [c] Ca-S = supplemented group calcium intake (mg); [d] Ca-effect = effect of Ca supplementation.

Vitamin D and fracture prevention: evidence of widespread vitamin D 'insufficiency' amongst population groups

The major source of vitamin D is the exposure of skin to the ultraviolet B-rays contained in sunlight. Of interest is the fact that in the UK there is no UV radiation of sufficient wavelength between October and March. It is now well established that vitamin D status is affected by the ageing process and the elderly population are of considerable concern with respect to the nutritional status of vitamin D and are clearly a group at risk of vitamin D 'insufficiency/deficiency'. For example, the findings of the National Diet and Nutritional Survey (NDNS) of people aged 65 years found 37% of those living in nursing homes had vitamin D deficiency (<25 nmol/l) and 97% of free-living elderly and 99% of nursing home residents had dietary intakes

Table 18.2 Calcium supplementation studies in late post-menopausal women. Data from New (1999).

Authors	Study duration (yrs)	n	Age (yrs)	TSM[a] (yrs)	Ca-C[b] (mg)	Ca-S[c] (mg)	Ca Effect[d]
Dawson-Hughes et al., 1995	2	169	60	> 5	283	783	+ve
Prince et al., 1995	2	168	63	> 10	787	1672	+ve
Reid et al., 1995	4	78	58	9	710	1570	+ve
Reid et al., 1993	2	122	58	9	730	1590	+ve
Nelson et al., 1991	2	36	60	11	761	1462	+ve
Dawson-Hughes et al., 1990	2	67	—	> 5	274	774	+ve

[a] TSM = time since menopause in years; [b] Ca-C = control group calcium intake (mg); [c] Ca-S = supplemented group calcium intake (mg); [d] Ca-effect = effect of Ca supplementation.

well below the RNI (mean intake ~ 2.5 µg) (Finch *et al.*, 1998). Of considerable surprise was the fact that similar trends were found in the more recent 2000 NDNS of young people aged 4–18 years (Gregory *et al.*, 2000). Quite clearly, these results have important implications for bone health and require an urgent focus of attention.

Vitamin D supplementation (with Ca) has been shown to be effective in reducing fracture rates in both institutionalised and free-living elderly populations, but vitamin D given as a supplement alone does not appear to be as effective. Furthermore, the level of vitamin D supplementation requires further attention. Studies which have been effective have used a level of between 17.5 and 20 µg/d whereas studies using only 10 µg/d have not resulted in a reduction in hip fracture incidence. Further studies are required to determine the exact level of vitamin D supplementation required for the prevention of fracture in the elderly.

Evidence of a positive link between fruit and vegetable intake and skeletal health?

Recent population-based studies suggest a positive association between high intakes of fruit and vegetables and bone health. The similarity of the findings of two of the largest (and most recent) nutrition and bone health surveys is a point of note (New *et al.*, 1997, 2000; Tucker *et al.*, 1999) (Table 18.3). The interpretation of these observation studies is con-

Table 18.3 Impact of fruit and vegetables on bone: a review of population-based studies showing a positive link.

Author	Year	Country	Details	Findings
Eaton-Evans *et al.*	1993	UK	77 Females, 46–56 Yrs	✓ vegetables
Michaelsson *et al.*	1995	Sweden	175 Females, 28–74 Yrs	✓ K intake
New *et al.*	1997	UK	994 Females, 45–49 Yrs	✓ K, Mg, fibre, vitamin C ✓ past intake of fruit and vegetable
New *et al.*	1998	UK	164 Females, 55–87 Yrs	✓ K, fruit and vegetables
Tucker *et al.*	1999	USA	229 Males, 349 Females, 75 Yrs	✓ K, Mg, fruit and vegetables
New *et al.*	2000	UK	62 Females, 45–54 Yrs	✓ K, Mg, fibre, vitamin C ✓ past intake of fruit and vegetable

Data from New (2000b). Reproduced with permission.

siderably strengthened by the reduction in urinary Ca excretion in the fruit and vegetable supplement group participating in the DASH intervention trial (Dietary Approaches to Stopping Hypertension) (Appel *et al.*, 1997). An increase in fruit and vegetable intake from 3.6 to 9.5 daily servings decreased urinary Ca from 157 mg/24hr to 110 mg/24hr. This is the first population-based fruit and vegetable intervention trial which showed (albeit as a secondary finding) a positive effect on Ca economy. The scientific community await with great interest the results of DASH II in which markers of both bone formation and resorption are being measured.

The link between fruit and vegetables and bone health may be explained by the growing recognition of the role of the skeleton in acid-base balance and the notable beneficial impact of an alkaline environment induced by a diet rich in fruit and vegetables. This is an exciting area for further research, the theoretical considerations of which have been discussed for over three decades (Barzel, 1970), but it has only recently received much further attention (New, 2000b).

Role of other micronutrients on bone health

There is growing interest in a link between vitamin K and bone health. Several vitamin K-dependent proteins, such as osteocalcin and matrix gla protein, are involved in bone mineralisation, and low circulating levels of vitamin K have been found in elderly and osteoporotic women. The publication of the first UK database on dietary vitamin K is of enormous benefit and will enable a much closer investigation of the impact of this nutrient on bone health to be determined in the near future (Bolton-Smith *et al.*, 2000).

The role of 'other' micronutrients (including magnesium, phosphorus, sodium, fluorine, trace elements (e.g. zinc, copper, manganese and boron), vitamin C and vitamin B) and 'other' dietary components (including alcohol, caffeine and phytoestrogens) on bone health remains relatively undefined. Data concerning their importance to the skeleton are sparse and the information that exists is from observational rather than intervention studies and subject numbers are often small.

Conclusion

The key points are:

- Predisposition to poor bone health, resulting in osteoporotic fracture, is a major public problem. Future economic impact will be phenomenal.
- Two mechanisms determine adult bone health: maximum attainment of PBM and postmenopausal bone loss. Both aspects are determined by a combination of endogenous and exogenous factors, with extensive interactions between them. As a modifiable factor, diet plays a vital role.
- There is considerable controversy concerning Ca and PBM development. The short-term effect appears beneficial but longer term results are questionable. There is evidence that Ca is effective in reducing late PBM bone loss but further work is required in perimenopausal women.
- Vitamin D (and Ca) have been shown to be effective in reducing fracture rates in the elderly population. There is evidence of widespread vitamin D 'insufficiency' in a number of population groups, which requires an urgent focus of attention.
- The possibility of a positive link between high fruit and vegetable consumption and bone health is an exciting 'new' area for further research.

- Our knowledge of the influence of other mironutrients remains limited. Further work is required to establish the essential ingredients for optimum bone health, particularly in those individuals who are genetically susceptible to osteoporosis.

References

Aloia, J.F., Vaswani, A., Yeh, J.K. *et al.* (1994) Calcium supplementation with and without hormone replacement therapy to prevent postmenopausal bone loss. *Ann. Int. Med.*, **120**, 97–103.

Appel, L.J., Moore, T.J., Obarzanek, E., Vallmer, W.M., Svetkey, L.P. Sacks, F.M., Bray, G.A., Vogt, T.M. & Cutler, J.A. (1997) A clinical trial of the effects of dietary patterns on blood pressure. *N. Eng. J. Med.*, **336**, 1117–24.

Barzel, U.S. (1970) The role of bone in acid-base metabolism. In: *Osteoporosis* (ed. U.S. Barzel), pp. 199–206. Grune & Stratton, New York.

Bolton-Smith, C., Price R.J.G., Fenton, S.T., Harrington, D.J. & Shearer, M.J. (2000) Compilation of a provisional UK database for the phylloquinone (vitamin K_1) contents of foods. *Brit. J. Nutr.*, **83**, 389–99.

Dawson-Hughes, B., Dallal, G.E., Krall, E.A., Sadowski, L., Sahyoun, N. & Tannerbaum, S. (1990) A controlled trial of the effect of Ca supplementation on bone density in postmenopausal women. *N. Eng. J. Med.*, **323**, 878–83.

Elders, P.J., Netelenbos, J.C., Lips, P. *et al.* (1991) Calcium supplementation reduces vertebral bone loss in perimenopausal women: a controlled trial in 248 women between 46 and 55 years of age. *J. Clin. End. Metab.*, **73**, 533–40.

Ettinger, B., Genant, H.K. & Cann, C.E. (1987) Postmenopausal bone loss is prevented by treatment with low-dosage oestrogen with calcium. *Ann. Intern. Med.*, **106**, 870–73.

Finch, S., Doyle, W., Lowe, C., Bates, C.J., Prentice, A., Smithers, G. & Clarke, P.C. (1998) *National Diet and Nutrition Survey: People Aged 65 Years and Over.* The Stationery Office, London.

Gregory, J., Lowe, S., Bates, C.J., Prentice, A., Jackson, L.V., Smithers, G., Wenlock, R. & Farron, M. (2000) *National Diet and Nutrition Survey (NDNS) of people aged 4-18 years*, vol. 1. The Stationery Office, London.

Nelson, M.E., Fisher, E.C. & Abraham Dilmanian, F.A. (1991) A 1-yr walking program and increased dietary calcium in postmenopausal women: effects on bone. *Am. J. Clin. Nutr.*, **53**, 1304–11.

New, S.A., Bolton-Smith, C., Grubb, D.A. & Reid, D.M. (1997) Nutritional influences on bone mineral density: a cross-sectional study in premenopausal women. *Am. J. Clin. Nutr.*, **65**, 1831–9.

New, S.A. (1999) Bone health: the role of micronutrients. *Br. Med. Bull.*, **55**, 619–33.

New, S.A., Robins, S.P., Campbell, M.K., Martin, J.C., Garton, M.J., Bolton-Smith, C., Grubb, D.A., Lee, S.J. & Reid, D.M. (2000) Dietary influences on bone mass and bone metabolism: further evidence of a positive link between fruit and vegetable consumption and bone health? *Am. J. Clin. Nutr.*, **71**, 142–51.

New, S.A. (2000a) Nutrition, exercise and bone health. *Proceedings of the Nutrition Society* (in press).

New, S.A. (2000b) Impact of food clusters on bone. In: *Nutritional Aspects of*

Osteoporosis 2000 (4th International Symposium on Nutritional Aspects of Osteoporosis, Switzerland) (eds B. Dawson–Hughes, P. Burckhardt & R.P. Heaney). *Challenges of Modern Medicine*. Ares-Serono Symposia Publications, Springer 2000 (in press).

Nilas, L., Borg, J., Gotfredsen, A. & Christiansen, C. (1984) *J. Nucl. Med.*, **26**, 1257-62.

Prince, R.L., Smith, M., Dick, I.M. *et al.* (1991) Prevention of postmenopausal osteoporosis: a comparative study of exercise, calcium supplementation and hormone-replacement therapy. *New Eng. J. Med.*, **325**, 1189-95.

Ralston, S.H. (1999) The genetics of osteoporosis. *Bone*, **25**, 85-6.

Reid, I.R., Ames, R.W., Evans, M.C. *et al.* (1993) Effect of calcium supplementation on bone loss in postmenopausal women. *New Eng. J. Med.*, **328**, 460-64.

Reid, I.R., Ames, R.W., Evans, M.C. *et al.* (1995) Long term effects of calcium supplementation on bone loss and fractures in postmenopausal women: A randomised controlled trial. *Am. J. Med.*, **98**, 331-5.

Riis, B., Thomsen, K. & Christiansen, C. (1987) Does calcium supplementation prevent postmenopausal bone loss? *New Eng. J. Med.*, **316**, 173-7.

Torgerson, D.J., Iglesias, C. & Reid, D.M. (2000) Economics of Osteoporosis. *Key Advance Series* (in press).

Tucker, K.L., Hannan, M.T., Chen, H., Cupples, A., Wilson, P.W.F. & Kiel, D.P. (1999) Potassium and fruit & vegetables are associated with greater bone mineral density in elderly men and women. *Am. J. Clin. Nutr.*, **69**, 727-36.

Weaver, C.M. (1999) Nutrition and bone health: the US perspective. *BNF Nutrition Bulletin*, **24**, 122-4.

World Health Organisation (1994). Assessment of fracture risk and its application to screening for osteoporosis. *Technical Series Report 843*. WHO, Geneva.

19

BEHAVIOUR CHANGE COUNSELLING

STEPHEN ROLLNICK & HAYLEY PROUT

Introduction

On the face of it, changing diet should be fairly straightforward. The choices involved do not approach the morale-sapping experience of severe hunger. Yet seemingly minor adjustments often acquire the status of major hurdles, as health care practitioners encounter the full weight of a patient's shopping and eating habits, personal preferences, anxiety, social rituals and cultural norms.

Healthcare practitioners also have their habits, perhaps none stronger than what could be called 'the righting reflex' (Miller & Rollnick, in press): if something is going wrong for a patient, it feels important to put things right. If this happens to be a poor diet, putting things right proves difficult however much we try to inform, advise or persuade patients. We are not social engineers and we cannot enter patients' lives and make the adjustments for them. Unlike many other healthcare interventions, encouraging lifestyle change is not just a matter of doing things *to* people. Beneath this rather simple observation lies the critical question: how does one encourage behaviour change in a patient? Is it just a matter of giving people expert-driven information?

This chapter will focus on the world of everyday healthcare rather than on the specialist field of eating disorders, since this is where most consultations about diet occur and where, by virtue of such large numbers, there is the greater potential for improving public health. The conclusion will amount to a paradox: in order to get better at changing patient behaviour we might first have to change our own – the way we approach these consultations and the skills we use to help people. Implications for practice, training and research will be highlighted.

What method?

Three broad approaches have been used within healthcare settings in the field of lifestyle change:

(1) Educational interventions (often brief advice)
(2) Behaviour change counselling
(3) Specialist therapies.

This chapter will focus on the second of these, which sits between the others in terms of complexity and suitability for different situations. Its rationale is derived from some dissatisfaction with the experience and effectiveness of educational interventions, and from the realisation that a wide range of healthcare practitioners can develop the skills required without immersing them in the jargon and complexity of specialist therapies. The evidence base for this is growing and some key skills can be identified, although there are clearly no 'quick-fix' counselling solutions to effecting change in others.

Educational interventions

Information overload?

The tendency to impart information about diet, both fearful and positive, pervades the media and healthcare practice. Even if the content of these messages were consistent, would they encourage change? Scrutiny of research on behaviour change suggests that information plays only a limited role when someone considers change. To maximise its impact, is it just a matter of what information is given to patients, or is there an art or a skill involved?

'Just do it, please'!

Persuading, imploring, warning and message-giving are widespread activities in talk with patients about behaviour change. Information-giving is seldom a benign activity when it comes to diet. It gets absorbed into advice-giving. The limitations of this activity are well known 'at the coal face' ('I keep telling them, but they never listen'). Advice-giving is even built into the fabric of healthcare itself: many a doctor will tell a patient, 'I'll refer you to the dietitian who will give you some advice and information about diet'.

When researchers examine the impact of brief lifestyle advice and information-driven programmes, the outcome appears positive. The accumulation of controlled trials is impressive, the evidence for implementation less so. Practitioners on the ground often seem wary about changing their routine practice in line with recommendations from research which often have a strong public health impetus (Rollnick *et al.*, 1999).

Specialist therapies

At the other end of the spectrum are specialist therapies, two good examples being cognitive-behaviour therapy and motivational interviewing, both of which address difficult behaviour change problems, but in different ways. While the former has largely remained within the specialist arena, with its own research base, the latter has been applied and evaluated in healthcare settings with an enthusiasm that verges on the reckless (Burke *et al.*, in press). Cognitive therapy is a structured and collaborative venture into the world of changing the way people think about their situation and their efforts to change it. Motivational interviewing (Miller & Rollnick, in press) is a form of counselling in which the client explores ambivalence about change, and the counsellor invites, not imposes, different perspectives compatible with the client's values.

There are clearly limits to the extent to which a method like motivational interviewing, based on the use of refined listening skills, can be packaged and delivered by practitioners without adequate training and time to spend with patients. In the case of cognitive-behaviour therapy, its specialist qualities might render it virtually inaccessible to generic healthcare practitioners (Durham *et al.*, 2000). Thus far, the home of these therapies is largely in the treatment by specialists of more severe problems like eating disorders.

Behaviour change counselling

We suggest that this term be used to describe the range of patient-centred methods that endorse the assumption that patients are best encouraged to be active decision-makers. This kind of counselling should not be confused with generic counselling, or other forms of counselling like bereavement counselling, because consultations about dietary or other lifestyle changes have a peculiar characteristic, a potential tension between the two parties over why and how change might be pursued, hence the oft-heard anecdote, '...the more I persuade, the harder they resist'.

Against a background of patient-centred research that appears to confirm the effectiveness of encouraging active decision-making (e.g. Greenfield *et al.*, 1988; Kaplan *et al.*, 1989), recent years have seen the emergence of a number of attempts to improve outcomes by utilising the stages of change model (Hunt & Hillsden, 1996) and adaptations of motivational interviewing (Rollnick *et al.*, 1999). The field of diabetes, for example, has seen a number of efforts to improve outcomes (see Burke *et al.*, in press; Resnicow *et al.*, in press) where diet has been a central focus. Attention here will be focused on methods themselves, since it is from this vantage point that practitioners, trainers and researchers should judge the utility of behaviour change counselling in the first instance. Some good examples of the breadth and scope of behaviour change counselling can be located in Hunt and Hillsden (1996). Illustrations here are derived more directly from adaptations of motivational interviewing, where it has been possible to refine a set of teachable skills that increase the flexibility of the practitioner's approach to behaviour change (Rollnick *et al.*, 1999).

The strategies below are ways of structuring a conversation about behaviour change in which the patient is encouraged to be as active as possible. Put another way, if you ask a patient, 'How do you feel about change?', these strategies are simply different ways of structuring the conversation that follows. The goal is to achieve shared decision-making. Sometimes patients who prefer to be passive recipients of the doctor's opinion can undermine this. So too, practitioners themselves often want to take control and convey their strong views about change to their patients. The rationale here is that it might be best to start a behaviour change consultation assuming that the patient would like to be more active in making decisions. If this is not the case this will soon become apparent. Similarly, if the practitioner has strong views about change, most patients will probably be more responsive if their own views are taken into account to begin with.

Information Exchange

This strategy is derived from motivational interviewing, from attempts to find out how best to help problem drinkers deal with the interpretation of wide-ranging test results. Apparently, motivation to change and actual outcome are enhanced if the patient, not the practitioner, interprets the personal relevance of test results (Burke *et al.*, in press). The practitioner first finds out what the patient knows and wants to know (*elicit*), then provides information in a neutral manner (*provide*), and finally draws out the patient's interpretation of its personal relevance (*elicit*) (see Rollnick *et al.*, 1999).

This framework is congruent with both the patient-centred model and research findings which support the hypothesis that an active, enquiring patient is more likely to improve on biomedical markers and in lifestyle change (Kaplan *et al.*, 1989). Practitioners often feel that they do not always have the time to do so much listening. However, used at key moments in the management of a condition or procedure, it might save time otherwise wasted in repeated messages that the patient apparently does not hear. Experience in training suggests that this framework is teachable, that it helps the practitioner to select what information to provide, but that its successful execution is dependent upon skilful listening in the first and third phases.

Agenda setting

If one has a choice of behaviours that could be targeted, how should one proceed? It is a daily challenge for practitioners in primary care, cardiovascular and pulmonary rehabilitation, pain management, diabetes and a number of other fields. The inclination to make choices for patients, by selecting which behaviour to focus on, runs against the hypothesis that patients are more likely to succeed if they select the behaviour and a target which they judge as suited to their circumstances. If a patient is more ready to change behaviour A than behaviour B, it would be unfortunate if the practitioner happened to focus first on behaviour B. Sometimes a practitioner might feel that change in behaviour B is more urgent, in which case a critical task is to negotiate an agenda to the satisfaction of both parties. One way of doing this is to make the choices explicit from the outset, allowing both parties to state their views before settling on a shared decision, for example:

> 'We could talk about change in your diet, getting more exercise or changing your tablets. What do you think about these possibilities, or would you prefer to be talking about something else?'

An early examination of this strategy was embodied in the agenda-setting chart used in a study of patients with chronic type 2 diabetes (Stott *et al.*, 1995; Pill *et al.*, 1998).

Among the lessons learned from this study, which failed to demonstrate an effect on hard outcomes, was that handing over some of the responsibility for decision-making to the patient is not easy for many practitioners; using this strategy is a skilful matter, with listening at the centre of the nego-tiation, the goal being to decide with the patient who should take responsibility for what, inside and outside the consulting room. It might be best targeted at newly-diagnosed patients with potentially chronic conditions.

Single behaviours: importance and confidence assessment

When talking to patients about a single, specific change in behaviour (e.g. taking more exercise, using a particular medication, stopping smoking), arguments for and against change emerge from the patient in the form of seemingly incompatible and irrational voices (e.g. 'I'd like to but I can't see me like that'). The skill required here is to avoid responding with counter-arguments, to adopt a more detached role, and to summarise one's understanding of the person's predicament. This in itself, can enhance motivation to change.

We developed a strategy for entering this terrain, 'assessing importance and confidence', in experimental consultations with smokers (Butler *et al.*, 1999). This pilot work and our review of the literature (Rollnick, 1998) led us to the conclusion that much of the model building in health psy-chology revolved around two central concepts: how *important* the change is for people (health beliefs, expectations of outcome) and how *confident* they feel about doing what is necessary to succeed (self-effi-cacy); or, put very simply, the *why* and *how* of change respectively. The interplay between these two concepts and readiness is illustrated in Figure 19.1. Put simply, high levels of importance and confidence will make for increased readiness to change.

The goal for the practitioner is to focus on the dimension of need. For example, to focus on confidence-building to get more exercise in a patient who is not convinced about its importance would be a mistake, highly likely to generate resistance and disengagement. To prevent this kind of mismatch, we developed a numerical assessment of these dimensions which practitioners used within the first minute or two of raising the subject of change. This provided a platform for either exploring importance or building confidence, with the patient being encouraged to drive the content of the discussion, aided by personally-tailored advice and information from the practitioner. Numerical and other strategies for structuring this process can be found in Rollnick *et al.* (1999).

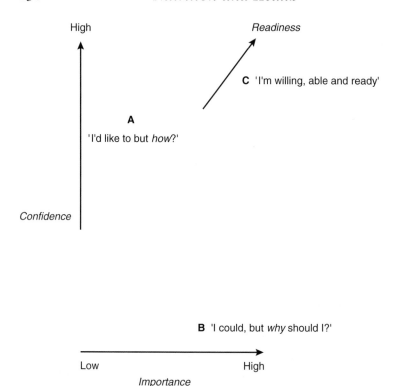

Figure 19.1   Importance, Confidence and Readiness: a practitioner's guide.

Awareness of these dimensions might be useful not just in lifestyle change consultations, but with any motivational problem encountered in every-day practice. For example, failure to take medication might occur because the patient does not share your understanding of the importance of the treatment plan, or because, as is common among elderly people, they lack confidence about remembering what tablets to take and when.

Some observations

The suggestion that this kind of activity is called behaviour change *counselling* is intended to discourage the view that behaviour change in patients can be achieved by applying one or more techniques *on* them. Both the stages of change model and motivational interviewing have proved vulnerable to this misunderstanding (Rollnick *et al.*, 1999). Counselling involves listening at its heart. While the above illustrations certainly involve structured and directed listening, no strategy or technique can provide a shortcut that avoids skilful listening.

Training in behaviour change counselling

If this form of counselling is within the grasp of healthcare practitioners, attention to training would appear paramount. It is difficult to escape the conclusion that in order to change patient behaviour, we might need to change our own first, i.e. learn new skills and widen our repertoire for dealing with behaviour change problems. In the first instance, practitioners need to address the 'righting reflex' and learn to restrain it. Helping the patient to be the expert involves a shift of responsibility in the consultation, and a shift in attitude for the practitioner that no amount of skill training can resolve. Once this more general attitude is absorbed, the practitioner is free to learn about listening skills and other aids to effective counselling.

Implifications for research

If research is to move beyond the evaluation of simpler educational interventions, it will be necessary to work within a more sophisticated evaluation framework. Behaviour change counselling and the more specialist methods are not like doses of medicine; they cannot be evaluated without careful monitoring of what happens inside the consultation. The training of practitioners, for example, cannot be viewed as a messy by-product of a more worthy endeavour, evaluating patient outcomes; it should form an essential early phase in the research process. Guidelines for evaluating complex interventions, like that produced by the Medical Research Council, are well worth following. Seen in this light, many of the controlled trials published to date have a decidedly premature feel to them (see Burke *et al.*, in press). Researchers have tended to ignore method development, careful training and adequate monitoring of the quality of interventions. We are therefore some distance from being able to establish whether more complex interventions like behaviour change counselling are effective, and under what circumstances.

Conclusion

In the field of lifestyle change, the subject of diet has proved particularly vulnerable to the lure of expert information, often delivered in a top-down manner to the passive patient. If it is the case that behaviour change for patients involves effort, confusion and vigilance, why are they so often rendered passive in the consulting room? This observation provides the rationale for behaviour change counselling: a patient who actively ponders the challenge of change in the consulting room is more likely to step outside and change. A practitioner who listens, supports, provides relevant information with skill, and who draws solutions from the patient, is more likely to be effective.

It is not difficult to tell the difference between crude and skilful bereavement counselling. For example, saying to a patient, 'Don't worry, you'll get over it' would be a good example of the former! So it is with behaviour change counselling. Patients have a right to expect practitioners to view them as individuals and to make some effort to understand their dilemmas and aspirations. The way they are spoken to is as important as the content of the information provided to them.

References

Burke, B., Arkowitz, H. & Dunn, C. (in press) The effectiveness of motivational interviewing and its adaptations: What we know so far. In: *Motivational Interviewing: Preparing People for Change*, 2nd edn (eds W. Miller & S. Rollnick). Guilford Press, New York.

Butler, C,. Rollnick, S., Cohen, D., Russell, I., Bachmann, M. & Stott, N. (1999) Motivational consulting versus brief advice for smokers in general practice: A randomized trial. *Brit. J. Gen. Pract.*, **49**, 611–16.

Durham, R., Swan, J. & Fisher, P. (2000) Complexity and collaboration in routine practice of CBT: what doesn't work with whom and how might it work better? *J. Mental Health*, **9**, 4429–44.

Greenfield, S., Kaplan, S.H., Ware, J.E., Yano, E.M. & Frank, H.J. (1988) Patients' participation in medical care: effects on blood sugar control and quality of life in diabetes. *J. Gen. Intern. Med.*, **3**, 448–57.

Hunt, P. & Hillsden, M. (1996) *Changing Eating and Exercise Behaviour*. Blackwell Science Ltd, Oxford.

Kaplan, S.H., Greenfield, S. & Ware, J.E. (1989) Assessing the effects of physician-patient interactions on the outcomes of chronic disease. *Med. Care*, **27**, S110–27.

Miller, W. & Rollnick, S. (in press) *Motivational Interviewing: Preparing People for Change*, 2nd edn. Guilford Press, New York.

Pill, R., Stott, N., Rollnick, S. & Rees, M. (1998) A randomised controlled trial of an intervention designed to improve the care given in general practice to Type II diabetic patients: patient outcomes and professional ability to change behavior. *Fam. Pract.*, **15**, 229–35.

Resnicow, K., Dilorio, C., Soet, J., Borrelli, B. & Hecht, J. (in press) Motivational interviewing in health promotion: It sounds like something is changing. In: *Motivational Interviewing: Preparing People for Change*, 2nd edn (eds W. Miller & S. Rollnick). Guilford Press, New York.

Rollnick, S. (1998) Readiness, importance and confidence: critical conditions of change in treatment. In: *Treating Addictive Behaviour*, 2nd edn. (eds W. R. Miller, N. Heather), Plenum, New York.

Rollnick, S., Mason, P. & Butler, C. (1999) *Health Behavior Change: A Guide for Practitioners*. Churchill Livingstone, Edinburgh.

Stott, N.C.H., Rollnick, S., Rees, M. & Pill, R. (1995) Innovation in clinical method: diabetes care and negotiating skills. *Fam. Pract.*, **12**, 413–18.

20

HEALTH CLAIMS – CAN THEY OFFER HOPE FOR CONSUMERS AS WELL AS 'HYPE' FOR INDUSTRY?

MARGARET ASHWELL

Consumer perception of benefit is equal to the true benefit plus the euphoria accompanying it (Ashwell, 1991). Claims about food products which relate to diet and health can only offer help, and hope, for consumers if the euphoria is in line with the benefit of the product. The job of the regulators is to provide a legal framework to control claims but scientists must provide a scientific basis for this framework. The role of the health professionals and the scientists is to help the consumer to disentangle the euphoria from the benefit. Without this input, some industry marketing departments will use claims purely as 'hype' for their products and consumer confusion will ensue. Put another way, the health professionals and scientists must act as the 'nits on the back of the marketing monkeys'! The nits must be more vigilant than ever now because of the enormous increase in the claims being made for 'functional foods'. 'Functional food' has become a buzz word in the food industry. Recent estimates suggest that the market for functional foods is approximately £830 million in Europe and it is predicted to jump to £1.6 billion by 2010 with the global value of this sector potentially equivalent to 5% of the world food market (Potter, 1999).

Authorisation of health claims

The concept of Foods for Specified Health Use (FOSHU) was established in Japan in 1991. These foods are included as one of the four categories of foods described in the Japanese Nutrition Improvement Law as 'foods for special dietary use' (i.e. 'foods that are used to improve people's health and for which specific health effects are allowed to be displayed'). Upon satisfactory submission of comprehensive data documenting the scientific evidence in support of a proposed health claim, the Minister of Health and Welfare is able to approve a claim, and grant permission, to use a 'symbol' on labelling, to indicate to the consumer that the health claim has government approval. Foods identified as FOSHU are required to provide evidence that the final food product is expected to exert a health or physiological effect; data on the effects of isolated individual components are not sufficient. FOSHU products should be in the form of ordinary foods (i.e. not as pills or capsules) and are assumed to be consumed as part of an ordinary diet (i.e. not as very occasional items linked to specific symptoms). Most FOSHU products currently approved contain either oligosaccharides or lactic acid bacteria for promoting intestinal health.

In the USA, 'reduction of disease risk' claims have been allowed since 1993 on certain foods. These contain components where the Food and Drug Administration (FDA) has accepted that there is objective evidence for a correlation between nutrients or foods in the diet and certain diseases on the basis of 'the totality of publicly available scientific evidence, and where there is substantial agreement amongst qualified experts that the claims were supported by the evidence'. By the end of 2000 there were 15 FDA-approved correlations between foods, or components, and diseases. The FDA also allows claims to be based on 'authoritative statements' of a Federal Scientific Body, such as the National Institutes of Health and Center for Disease Control as well as from the National Academy of Sciences, as allowed by the FDA Modernization Act of 1997 (two of the fifteen health claims have been allowed under the this Act). The FDA is now considering a process whereby a company can apply to the FDA in respect of a particular nutrition and health link they wish to claim. The company would fund studies to develop evidence for their proposed claim and the FDA would 'direct' this research to monitor its quality. The FDA have published a document as *Guidance for Industry* which contains scientific principles for those designing studies to support health claims petitions (US Food and Drug Administration, 1999). This is a very useful document which covers identifying data for review, performing reliable measurements, evaluating individual studies, evaluating the totality of the evidence and assessing significant scientific agreement.

In the European Union, there is no harmonised legislation on health claims which means that they are dealt with at a national level. Not surprisingly, there have already been several calls for better regulation of functional and health claims for foods and supplements (Katan, 1999). It is therefore up to scientists and health professionals to ensure that a proper scientific basis for these claims is established as soon as possible.

What are functional foods?

The recent consensus document on scientific concepts of functional foods in Europe (FUFOSE) (Diplock *et al.*, 1999) was an important development in this area. Key definitions from the document are as follows:

- A food can be regarded as 'functional' if it is satisfactorily demonstrated to affect beneficially one or more target functions in the body, beyond adequate nutritional effects in a way which is relevant to either an improved state of health and well-being and/or reduction of risk of disease. Functional foods must remain foods and they must demonstrate their effects in amounts which can normally be expected to be con- sumed in the diet. They are not pills or capsules, but part of a normal food pattern.
- A functional food can be a natural food, a food to which a component has been added, or a food from which a component has been removed by technological or biotechnological means. It can also be a food where the nature of one or more components has been modified, or a food in which the bioavailability of one or more components has been modified, or any combination of these possibilities. A functional food might be functional for all members of a population or for particular groups of the population which might be defined, for example, by age or by genetic constitution.

However, the main thrust of the consensus document (Diplock *et al.*, 1999) was to suggest a novel scheme whereby claims for functional foods should be linked to solid scientific evidence, based on markers.

Types of nutrition and health claims

In 1999 Codex Alimentarius (1999) proposed draft recommendations for the use of health claims and identified two types of claims. 'Enhanced function claims' concern specific beneficial effects of the consumption of foods and their constituents on physiological (or psychological) functions or biological activities but do not include nutrient function claims. Such claims relate to a positive contribution to health or to a condition linked to health, to the improvement of a function or to modifying or preserving health. 'Reduction of disease risk claims' are 'for reduction of disease risk

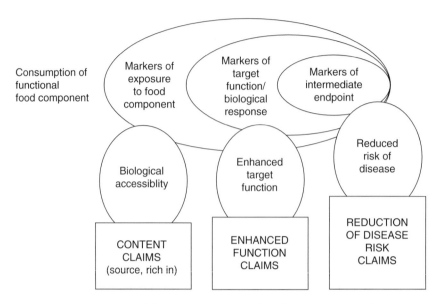

Figure 20.1 A proposal for a scientific basis for all claims (Ashwell, 2001).

related to the consumption of a food or food constituent in the context of the daily diet that might help reduce the risk of a specific disease or condition'. Although amendments to these definitions are the subject of consultation, the distinction between the two types of claims is still preserved (Codex Alimentarius, 2000).

The Codex proposals bear a pleasing congruence with the type A (enhanced function claims) and type B (reduced risk of disease claims) suggested in the consensus document (Diplock *et al.*, 1999), which proposed that claims should be based on evidence related to markers which are linked to clearly defined and measurable outcomes and are significantly and consistently modulated in rigorously controlled studies by the particular food component.

Enhanced function claims should be accompanied by evidence based on valid, reproducible, sensitive and specific markers relating to the target function or biological response, such as changes in body fluid levels of a metabolite, protein or enzyme (e.g. the reduction in levels of plasma homocysteine as a response to dietary folate, or the increased levels of brain serotonin as a response to dietary tryptophan).

Reduction of disease risk claims, however, would only be justified if the evidence is based on valid, reproducible, sensitive and specific markers relating to an appropriate intermediate endpoint of an improved state of health and well-being and/or reduction of risk of disease, such as the measurement of a biological process which relates directly to the end-point (e.g. the extent of narrowing of the carotid artery as evidence of cardiovascular disease; or functional imaging of the brain by magnetic resonance imaging as an intermediate endpoint marker for the amelioration of depression).

This suggestion that the type of claim made should relate to the type of marker was indeed a novel approach to the evaluation of the scientific support for health-related claims for foods and food components. The FDA document (US Food and Drug Administration, 1999) gives guidance on which acceptable biomarkers can be used to support health claims but it does not go further than this.

The new Codex proposals, if accepted, will ultimately be incorporated into the existing Codex general guidelines on claims where four different types of nutrition claims have already been defined. One of these is the nutrient content claim which refers to the level of a nutrient contained in a food, such as 'source of calcium' or 'rich in folic acid'. At present, there is UK legislation to ensure that nutrient content claims for vitamins and minerals are only made if the food contains a significant amount of micronutrient in relation to its recommended daily allowance ('labelling' RDA) (Statutory Instruments, 1996). There has never been a requirement to show that the nutrient in the food actually is biologically accessible to the body and it has always been assumed that any additional nutrient which might be added as a fortificant behaves in the same way as the nutrient found naturally in the food.

Biological accessibility

To a small extent the existing legislation for vitamins and minerals takes biological accessibility into account because RDAs are recommendations of intakes which are calculated from knowledge of population requirements and the average bioavailability of that nutrient in 'normal' foods. However, very little evidence exists for the biological accessibility of vitamins and minerals in fortified foods, let alone other potential components in functional foods such as isoflavonoids. If all claims are to have a scientific base, then it should not be enough just to state that a functional food contains a certain amount of a food component. The biological accessibility of that component within that functional food should be demonstrated. In the case of functional food components which are purported to act intracellularly, this will require the demonstration of absorption of the functional food component through the intestinal wall at least into the bloodstream. In the case of functional food components which act within the gut, this would require the demonstration of their presence at the site of action.

If the logic from The EC Concerted Action on Functional Food Science in Europe is extended to its extreme, then my personal view is that the same scientific logic should extend to 'nutrient content' claims, particularly if applied to 'novel' functional food components (Ashwell, 2001). These should be based not only on evidence of presence of the component in the food, but also on scientific evidence using markers of exposure which indicate the biological accessibility of the active component such as its delivery to the intestine or its absorption through the intestinal wall and into the relevant cells, as appropriate. My proposal (as summarised in Figure 20.1 on p 142) is an extension to the FUFOSE scheme and it offers a simple scientific framework for the preparation of 'support dossiers', as well as a broad framework for the regulation of *all* claims (nutrient claims and health claims).

The difference between the potential European scheme and my refinement of it and the system for regulating health claims in USA is best illustrated with the example of a recently allowed FDA health claim for the beneficial effect of soya protein on cardiovascular disease. On the basis of the scientific evidence available, the FDA concluded that one of the model statements that can be made is as follows:

> 25 g of soy protein a day, as part of a diet low in saturated fat and cholesterol, may reduce the risk of heart disease.

The potential European scheme would not, however, on the basis of the current scientific evidence, allow this 'reduction of disease risk' claim to be made, but would consider that the evidence would only justify an 'enhanced function' claim'. This might be along the lines of 'helps maintain healthy arteries' because as yet there is no direct evidence for soy protein reducing, say, the narrowing of carotid arteries (see Figure 20.2).

At the time of pronouncing on the soy protein claim, the FDA were not convinced that the isoflavones were the active component of soy in terms of lowering LDL-cholesterol. However, there is a lot of excitement about the beneficial effects of isoflavones from soy and many manufacturers are

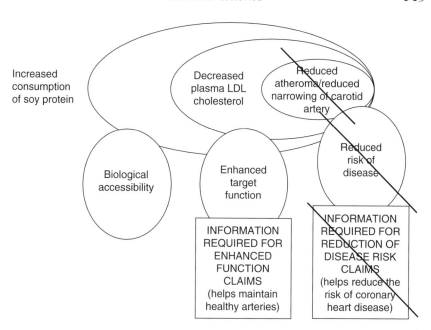

Figure 20.2 The scientific basis for claims for 'functional' food components – example of a soy protein as a functional food component.

now selling isoflavone supplements. Content claims such as 'rich source of isoflavones' are becoming very common and the more responsible manufacturers state the amount of isoflavones in their product. But a recent analysis of 20 isoflavone supplements (Setchell *et al.*, 2001) has drawn attention to considerable differences in the isoflavone content compared with that claimed by the manufacturer. Moreover, plasma iso-flavone concentrations showed marked qualitative and quantitative dif-ferences depending on which supplement is ingested. Thus a scheme for checking the biological accessibility of a food component before allowing a claim (as shown in Figure 20.3) would make it harder for less responsible manufacturers to make a claim for a non-biologically effective food com-ponent.

Conclusion

The general scheme in Figure 20.1 is intended to be used in conjunction with codes of practice, such as the Joint Health Claims Initiative (JHCI) in the UK, which cover the issues of evaluating the totality of the evidence and assessing significant scientific agreement. Health professionals should

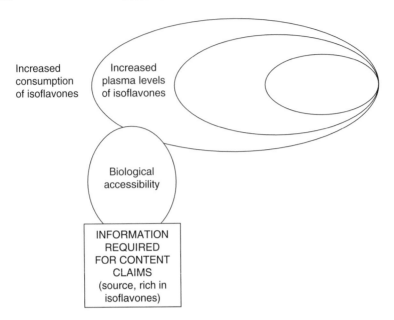

Figure 20.3 The scientific basis for claims for 'functional' food components – example of a isoflavones as a functional food component.

encourage and help the food industry to think along these lines. Not only will this help the industry to gain a good reputation for making truthful claims rather than using them for 'hype', it will also help to preserve a good reputation for the science of nutrition and the people who work within it. If the same people can also play an important role in educating consumers or advising the people who educate consumers, then a consistent message will be promulgated. This must be a long term objective for improving public health and for giving consumers confidence and hope.

References

Ashwell, M. (2001) Functional foods: a simple scheme for establishing the scientific basis for all claims. *Public Health Nutrition*, **4** (3), 859–62.

Ashwell, M.A. (1991) Consumer perception of food related issues. *BNF Nutrition Bulletin*, **16**, 25–35.

Codex Alimentarius (1999) *Proposed draft recommendations for the use of health claims*. WHO, Geneva.

Codex Alimentarius (2000) *Proposed draft guidelines for the use of health and nutrition claims*. WHO, Geneva.

Diplock, A., Aggett, P. *et al.* (1999) Scientific Concepts of Functional Foods in Europe: Consensus Document. *Brit. J. Nutr.*, **81**, S1–S27.

Katan, M. (1999) Functional foods. *Lancet*, **354**, 794.

Potter, D (1999) Total integration. *Functional Foods and Nutraceuticals*, **2**, 30–32.

Setchell, K., Brown, N. *et al.* (2001) Bioavailability of isoflavones in healthy humans and analyses of commercial soy isoflavone supplements. *J. Nutr.*(in press).

Statutory Instruments (1996) *The Food Labelling Regulations*, SI No. 1499 of 1996. HMSO, London.

US Food and Drug Administration (1999) *Guidance for Industry Significant Scientific Agreement in the Review of Health Claims for Conventional Foods and Dietary Supplements.*

21

THE ROLE OF THE MEDIA

GEOFF WATTS

What is the role of the media in nutrition and health? Specifically, none at all. In general terms the media exist to report, reflect, comment, entertain and sometimes persuade. They certainly discuss nutrition and health, as they do everything else. But to say the media 'have a role' in nutrition and health is misleading. It implies some kind of pre-ordained duty to take on certain specific educational tasks decided by some (doubtless well-meaning) central authority charged with ensuring that press, radio and television do their bit for the greater good, play their part in a well-ordered society, and are prevented from upsetting the apple cart too often. The reality is not like this, and anything which creates such an impression is misleading.

In practice, of course, the media can and do disseminate useful information about health and nutrition. How? Self-evidently by doing those five things already mentioned: reporting, reflecting, commenting, entertaining and persuading. The media talk to the experts, then to their readers, listeners and viewers – or they provide opportunities for experts themselves to communicate directly with the public.

Agendas

The difficulty is that the parties involved in this enterprise are not always singing from the same hymn sheet or following an identical agenda. Factual inaccuracy in the media is not usually the biggest problem in the relationships with those professionals on whose activities they report; differing agendas are more often a source of conflict and disagreement.

What do doctors, scientists and nutritionists want from the media? To see reports of what they consider the most valuable developments and the most important messages. What do commercial organisations want? To see sympathetic accounts of their various products and activities. What do the media want? To be read, listened to, or watched by as many people as possible.

Sometimes these agendas coincide; often they do not. The media are not a social service; they exist to make a profit, and making a profit depends on being noticed. Even the BBC is not free of 'commercial' pressures; if it has no audience, it cannot justify the licence fee.

In short, what is important to doctors and nutritionists (i.e. what furthers their interest in the attainment of good health through better eating), and what might be good for consumers (eating what the experts say is the ideal diet) are not necessarily what is important to journalists (i.e. what gets read and listened to). Many people in medicine and science are still genuinely puzzled to discover that their view of what should be reported is not automatically accepted by the press.

This is not to suggest that journalism should have a licence for irresponsible reporting, or that journalists should not think about the consequences of what they say and write. Some do all the time, a few do none of the time, and most try to most of the time. Nor is it the case that things could not be different in the best of all possible worlds. The point is that to change anything you have to have a realistic perception of the way things are now. If people in science and medicine view the media as nothing more than a free and easy means of disseminating their particular views, they are going to be sorely disappointed.

Some pitfalls

Reporting new facts out of context

Science advances on a broad front; the media, especially in news bulletins, often report on single, isolated pieces of evidence. For example, micronutrients, phytoprotectants, soya, calcium supplementation and allergies have each been discussed at this meeting. Each is a perfectly legitimate topic for study, and with something to contribute to health. But articles or programmes in recent years have given the impression that each of these is a panacea. Do this, do that and you will solve such and such a problem. This fragmentation is endemic in the way the media work.

This presents a real difficulty for the conscientious journalist, because if the facts truly are put in context, the story may simply disappear! There is a fine balance to be struck between selling a story hard enough to get the reader's or listener's attention – but not so hard that it becomes hyped out of all reason.

Disseminating disagreement and spreading uncertainty

At various times, coffee has been associated with all sorts of ailments – not just the most familiar, heart disease, but various cancers, psychological disturbances and, recently, rheumatoid arthritis.

The link between coffee and heart disease, or more often coffee and cholesterol level, has been the subject of various findings over the years. Some researchers have found stronger links than others; some have found no link at all. There has also been the question of whether real or instant coffee is better or worse.

There are many other examples: fat and breast cancer; alcohol and heart disease; oils, fats and heart disease; even dietary fibre. Successive pieces of evidence appear to confirm, then disprove, then reconfirm the links.

All these findings are reported by the media. But what are readers, listeners and viewers to make of them? The fundamental difficulty is that few people understand that in science all findings are provisional. Its very basis is re-examination and, not infrequently, change. Reporting such changes often confuses the public; people wrongly view the word 'scientific' as meaning 'definitive' rather than simply 'the best explanation currently to hand'. The media (often unfairly) get the blame for upsetting the public when they are simply reporting what has happened.

The result is confusion. People view these developments not as the normal operation of science, but its failure – and this tends to undermine their trust in science as a whole.

What to do

To some extent there is no remedy. Certain of the problems are structural: a reflection of the differing natures and purposes of science and the media. But a few precautions may minimise the risk of disaster.

Openness and transparency: 'experts' who do not know should say they do not know – particularly in the context of safety questions. When quoting statistics for risk, these should be put in terms that people are most likely to be familiar with: the chance of being struck by lightening, run over by a car, whatever.

Enthusiasm for the topic in question when dealing with journalists is a valuable asset – provided the individual being questioned or interviewed does not try to oversell the findings. It is easy to be pushed into seeming to make stronger claims than originally intended. At all costs avoid retreating into jargon, even if it feels more comfortable than using simple, non-technical English.

Things will still, from time to time, go wrong. But people who have followed these and similar precautions will at least know they have done their best: a valuable comfort if not a foolproof shield against blame. The most important thing to remember is that the media are setting out to meet their own needs, and only incidentally those of the people on whose activities they report. The art of working with them lies in finding the common ground where agendas can mesh: the experts get the essence of their message across and the media get their story. Sometimes it does happen.

22

PRIMARY HEALTH CARE PROFESSIONALS – WORKING TOGETHER IN THE COMMUNITY

JUDY BUTTRISS

Over the past year or so, government has issued various documents which together provide a framework for delivering public health nutrition advice and information, and related lifestyle messages such as those focusing on physical activity, to the public. These publications include: the strategy document *Saving Lives: Our Healthier Nation* (DoH, 1999a); *The NHS Plan: a plan for investment, a plan for reform* (DoH, 2000a); *The NHS Cancer Plan* (DoH, 2000b); and *The National Service Framework for Coronary Heart Disease* (DoH, 2000c). During this period there have been other strategy documents that are also of relevance, e.g. *Sport in Education* published in 2000 (see Sport England website for details: www.sportengland.com). Coupled with this are ongoing campaigns such as that concentrating on folic acid, targeting women of child bearing age with a view to decreasing the prevalence of NTD-affected pregnancies (DoH, 2000d).

This chapter summarises the recommendations and requirements made by these documents and the challenges and opportunities they offer health care professionals working in the community.

Our Healthier Nation

Saving Lives: Our Healthier Nation set two targets of relevance to nutrition, to be achieved by the year 2010:

- Cancer – to reduce the death rate in people under 75 years by at least a fifth
- Coronary heart disease and stroke – to reduce the death rate in people under 75 years by at least two-fifths.

Targets were also set for accidents and mental health. Many were surprised by the absence of targets for weight management and obesity, or even for tackling physical inactivity, given that there has been an unabated increase in the prevalence of these conditions over recent decades. More than one in two British adults (62% of men and 53% of women) are overweight (a body mass index (BMI), > 25 kg/m^2), including one in five (17% of men and 21% of women) who are clinically obese (BMI > 30 kg/m^2) (DoH, 1999b). This represents a dramatic change since 1980 when 6% of men and 8% of women were obese. It has been estimated that, since 1970, daily energy intake has fallen by about 20% (Prentice & Jebb, 1995), whereas obesity has increased substantially over this time and people have become less active. The prevalence of obesity has increased by 50% among men in the last 10 years and by 42% in women (Petersen *et al.*, 1999).

A key emphasis of the *Our Healthier Nation* strategy document is the need to tackle health inequalities, i.e. the need to improve the health of everyone but the health of the worst off in particular. This follows on from the work of the Low Income Project Team, which was part of the previous government's *The Health of the Nation* initiative (DoH, 1992) and the *Independent Inquiry into Inequalities in Health* (Acheson, 1998).

Unlike its predecessor, the initiative known as *The Health of the Nation* (DoH, 1992), the *Our Healthier Nation* strategy document does not contain any specific nutrition targets, however it does promote the concept of a healthy and balanced diet (as depicted in the Balance of Good Health, otherwise known as the plate model), and it does emphasise the importance of physical activity. In terms of the latter, the document stresses that failure to reach the recommended levels of physical activity (30 minutes of moderate activity five times per week) doubles risk of coronary heart disease and triples risk of suffering a stroke. The risk of coronary heart disease in sedentary people is twice that of active people, and 60% of men and 70% of women can be classed as sedentary. Consequently, the population attributable risk of physical inactivity is very high.

The document also emphasises the role for public health nutritionists in achieving the objectives of the strategy, public health nutrition being focused on promotion of good health and the primary prevention of diet-related illness, via food and nutrition (and lifestyle change). Public health nutrition emphasises the maintenance of *wellness* in the whole population, although it may also include identifying and working with high risk and other groups within the population. Again, this emphasis is not new, and the Nutrition Society has already put in place a scheme for registering individuals with competence in public health nutrition (RPHNutr. – Registered Public Health Nutritionist) and a mechanism for encouraging high standards in the training of public health nutritionists via a course accreditation process (details at website: www.nutsoc.org.uk).

Our Healthier Nation also heralded new initiatives and bodies, such as the Health Development Agency, which is focusing on the need for an evidence-based approach, and the need to set standards for public health and health promotion practice. It is recognised that the public health workforce needs to be appropriately skilled, and a major barrier to delivery of targets is the absence of a multi-disciplinary basis to public health and its practice. Initiatives targeting the health of children have also been put in place. For example, Sure Start, which is a cross-governmental programme for parents and local communities, and the Healthy Schools programme, which embraces Cooking for Kids, the Safer Travel to School scheme, and Wired for Health which is a website for schools to help young people make informed decisions.

Our Healthier Nation also focuses on the need for partnerships and announces the reorienting of local services (including the NHS). It also stresses the strategic role for health authorities within the local partnerships that will be required in order to deliver the strategy, i.e. local health improvement programmes (HImPs). These will comprise locally determined priorities and targets, with an emphasis on health inequalities and with rewards to health authorities that make the best progress. These plans are elaborated in the National Service Framework for CHD (DoH, 2000c). Other developments include Health Action Zones and Healthy Living Centres.

The NHS Plan

The NHS Plan, launched in summer 2000, develops the theme of partnerships and has set targets in this context. By 2002 there will be new integrated public health groups across NHS regional offices and regional government offices, accountable through the regional Director of Public Health. By 2002 there will also be a new Healthy Communities Collaborative to spread best practice, and by 2003 there will be a leadership programme for health visitors and community nurses.

The NHS Plan includes some specific diet and health targets, to be delivered by 2004:

- A national school fruit scheme for every child in nursery education and 4–6 year olds at school. Pilots are now underway and the expectation is that the scheme will be rolled out towards the end of 2001.
- A 5-a-day national campaign to encourage fruit and vegetable consumption.
- The intention to work with industry (producers and retailers) to improve access and provision of fruit and vegetables.
- Also to work with industry, alongside the Food Standards Agency, to tackle the salt, fat and sugar content of the national diet.
- Development of a hospital nutrition policy, with the objective of decreasing the dependency on intravenous feeding and increasing the quality of foods in hospital.
- Action to reduce overweight and obesity, and to increase physical activity, by linking with the work of the Health Development Agency on assessing effective interventions for local action.

To help ensure a healthy start to life, by 2004 the NHS Plan proposes to deliver:

- Expansion of the Sure Start programme to cover a third of all children aged under 4 years living in poverty (to help break the cycle of deprivation).
- Reform of the welfare foods programme, to enable more effective use of resources for low income families and to provide more support for breastfeeding and parenting.
- Full implementation of the teenage pregnancy strategy published by the Social Exclusion Unit in 1999.

The NHS Plan is not the only document to highlight the need for action in these areas. For instance, the Malnutrition Advisory Group (MAG) launched its guidelines for detection and management of malnutrition at the end of November 2000. Undernutrition is frequently unrecognised and untreated in the community, in hospitals (in-patients and out-patients), and in nursing homes. MAG has developed a tool which can be used by health professionals in the community to identify and treat poor nutrition in adults.

National Service Framework for CHD

This series of documents sets various standards (DoH, 2000c). The relevant ones here are those that apply to the population at large (Standards 1 and 2) and those that apply to the primary prevention of cardiovascular disease in at-risk patients (Standards 3 and 4). Standard 12 concerns secondary prevention. These standards set challenges for community health care professionals and will be delivered via the HImPs mentioned above. Standard 1 states that the NHS and partner agencies should develop, implement and monitor policies that reduce the prevalence of coronary risk factors in the population, and reduce inequalities in risks of developing heart disease. Standard 2 states that the NHS and partner agencies should contribute to a reduction in the prevalence of smoking in the local population. Standard 3 states that GPs and primary care teams should identify all people with established cardiovascular disease and offer them comprehensive advice and appropriate treatment to reduce their risks. To meet Standard 4, all GPs and primary care teams should identify all people at significant risk of cardiovascular disease but who have not yet developed symptoms and offer them appropriate advice and treatment to reduce their risk.

Milestones have been set for the achievement of these standards. For example, in relation to Standards 1 and 2, by April 2001 all NHS bodies (working closely with local authorities) should have agreed and be delivering the local programme of effective policies. The latter is expected to target bringing about a reduction in smoking, promotion of healthy eating, promotion of physical activity, and reducing the prevalence of overweight and obesity. HImPs are to act as the vehicle for developing the partnerships and delivering the effective policies. The document specifies that the healthy eating programme should stress the need for a balanced diet with emphasis on the need to eat more fruit and vegetables, fish (especially oily fish), and starchy foods such as bread, rice, pasta and potatoes, and which includes a smaller proportion of foods containing fat and saturates, and less salt. It adds that 'consumption of moderate quantities of alcohol is unlikely to do harm and there may be some benefit', but notes that habitual and excessive alcohol consumption (about 4 units per day) can raise blood pressure. Attention is drawn to resources such as the Balance of Good Health, Guidelines for Educational Materials for School, Guidelines on Hospital Catering, and Eating Well at School.

NHS Cancer Plan

The NHS Cancer Plan (DoH, 2000b) emphasises smoking as the major factor that needs to be addressed from a lifestyle perspective, but adds that 'what people eat is the next biggest contributor to cancer deaths'. Particular emphasis is given to the need to eat more fruit and vegetables. As mentioned earlier, the government is working on various schemes to enhance fruit and vegetable consumption. The document also draws attention to the need to tackle obesity, physical inactivity and alcohol intake in the context of cancer prevention. Again, various milestones have been set. The 2000 targets include publication of Health Development Agency guidance on effective interventions (smoking, diet, physical activity and obesity) (HDA, 2000), and for pilots to begin for the National School Fruit Scheme and the local 5-a-day schemes. By 2001, the Plan calls for local action to be in place to address diet, physical activity and obesity, and the roll out of the School Fruit Scheme. From 2002 onwards, we can expect a roll out of the 5-a-day initiatives.

Effective interventions

The use of effective interventions will be a key component in achieving these ambitious targets. The Heath Education Authority (now the Heath Development Agency) has been assessing the outcomes of various types of local intervention, and has now published guidance (HDA 2000). By this mechanism, the main characteristics of effective healthy eating interventions have been identified as:

- Focus on diet alone, or diet and physical activity
- Set goals that are clear and are based on theories of behaviour change rather than information alone
- Involve personal contact over a sustained period with individuals or in a small group
- Provide feedback to participants
- Promote changes in the local environment, e.g. catering outlets
- Are developed around barriers to dietary change in the local community and work at several levels.

Similarly, effective physical activity interventions (Hillsden *et al.*, 1999; HDA, 2000) are:

- The use of home-based programmes, including those that could be carried out from home, e.g. walking

- Frequent professional contact
- Schools initiatives linked with external support services
- Moderate intensity activity, e.g. brisk walking
- Walking as the promoted mode of exercise
- Modifications to the environment, e.g. signposting to stairs.

With all of these approaches, it is important to consider the needs of the target groups. In the National Service Framework for CHD there is a specific recommendation to develop local strategies that link primary care teams with local authorities, e.g. exercise referral programmes (DoH, 2000c).

Characteristics of effective weight reduction interventions (HDA, 2000) include:

- Reduce sedentary behaviour in children
- Involve family therapy to prevent weight regain in children, rather than conventional diet and exercise protocols
- Use diet, physical activity and behavioural strategies, in combination, in adults
- Adopt a gradual, incremental, step-wise approach
- Acknowledge that potential barriers may include lack of access to appropriate support services or lack of motivation by professionals
- Be aware of the higher prevalence in more deprived groups, which needs to be considered when planning services.

A useful reference on obesity has been produced by the British Nutrition Foundation (BNF, 1999) and early in 2000, *Tackling Obesity* was published by the Faculty of Public Health Medicine (Maryon Davis *et al.*, 2000). This is a useful practical resource designed for use in the community.

Conclusions

These various government initiatives address many but not all of the important nutrition subjects covered in this book. Although no targets exist for obesity reduction, it is now being emphasised as an important issue to be addressed at local level through the activities of HImPs; time will tell if this approach is sufficient to stem this increasing problem. Many obese people are also diabetic. Diabetes is also on the government's agenda and a National Service Framework addressing this issue is expected in 2001. Although none of the documents highlight the importance of folic acid in early pregnancy, this presumably remains an important policy strand which health care professionals need to incorporate within their work. Similarly, there is a need for professionals to be alert to the need to address malnutrition in the community (MAG, 2000).

Although the importance of a varied and balanced diet underpins the dietary advice offered by government, many of the initiatives underway focus on fruit and vegetable consumption. This approach has the advantage that it is a positive message and its impact can be evaluated relatively easily compared with the delivery of the complex messages related to fat reduction, but is this approach going to lead to overall improvements in nutrient intake, given that many of the nutrients shown to be present in inadequate amounts in the diets of older school children (Buttriss, 2000; Gregory *et al.*, 2000) and older adults (Buttriss, 1999) are not present in large amounts in these foods (see Table 22.1), e.g. iron, calcium, zinc and riboflavin? It remains to be seen whether a focus on fruit and vegetable consumption, specifically, will lead to increases in the overall nutrient provision of the diet through general improvements in dietary balance, i.e. beneficial changes in the consumption of foods that provide the micronutrients not present in high concentrations in fruit and vegetables. Perhaps the pilots already underway may help throw light on this question.

Table 22.1 Proportion of 11–18 year olds with intakes of selected micronutrients below the lower reference nutrient intake (LRNI) (Gregory *et al.*, 2000).

	11–14 years		15–18 years	
	Boys %	Girls %	Boys %	Girls %
Iron		45		50
Calcium	12	24	9	19
Zinc	14	37	9	10
Magnesium	28	51	18	53
Riboflavin	6	22	6	21

An issue not addressed to any great extent by the Health Development Agency is the nature of the message. It is generally agreed that it is more productive to talk about foods than nutrients, but can people deal with several messages, e.g. eat more fruit and vegetables *and* reduce intake of fat-rich foods, particularly when one message is positive (eat more) and the other negative (eat less)? Also, what is the best approach when it comes to folate and folic acid – the mix of a food message and a supplement message?

No doubt health care professions have been set some tough challenges. *Our Healthier Nation* acknowledges that skills acquisition is crucial if the required healthy eating messages are to be delivered effectively. Wrong or incomplete advice is probably worse than no advice at all. It causes confusion at the very least, can result in apathy – 'they keep changing their minds' – and at worst can do harm. All those who engage in the provision of advice on nutrition have a professional responsibility personally to ensure that the advice they offer is sound and relevant, evidence-based, up-to-date and consistent, and will not do harm. It is recommended that all health professionals receive some training in basic nutrition and that this is modelled on the Core Curriculum for Health Professionals, published by the Department of Health in 1994. The Core Curriculum focuses on three areas: principles in nutrition science, public health nutrition, and clinical and nutritional support.

The Health Development Agency suggests that it may be worth considering ring fencing a block of time to enable in-service training to be provided by a community dietitian. Others in the community that can help with updating nutritional knowledge are public health nutritionists (RPHNutr.) To be registered with the Nutrition Society, public health nutritionists need an appropriate academic training and a minimum of 3 years' relevant experience post-graduation (details can be found at the Society's website: www.nutsoc.org.uk). The Heath Development Agency stresses the value of using local people to complement the work of health professionals. This approach can help establish self-reliance and community participation, and helps to overcome barriers to change that may exist locally.

References

Acheson, D. (1998) *Independent Inquiry into Inequalities in Health*. The Stationery Office, London.

BNF (1999) British Nutrition Foundation. *Obesity: the Report of the British Nutrition Foundation Task Force*. Blackwell Science, Oxford.

Buttriss, J. (1999) Nutrition in older people. Public Health Message. *BNF Nutrition Bulletin*, **24**, 48–57.

Buttriss, J. (2000) Diet and nutritional status of 4–18 year-olds: public health implications. *BNF Nutrition Bulletin*, **25**, 209–17.

DoH (1994) *Nutrition: core curriculum for nutrition in the education of health professionals*. Report produced as part of The Health of the Nation initiative. The Department of Health, London.

DoH (1992) *The Health of the Nation – a Strategy for Health in England*. The Stationery Office, London.

DoH (1999a) *Saving Lives: Our Healthier Nation*. The Stationery Office, London.

DoH (1999b) *Health Survey for England: Adults Reference tables '99 - obesity figures*. London: Department of Health (website: www.doh.gov.uk).

DoH (2000a) *The NHS Plan: a plan for investment, a plan for reform*. The Stationery Office, London.

DoH (2000b) *The NHS Cancer Plan*. Department of Health, London.

DoH (2000c) *The National Service Framework for Coronary Heart Disease*. Department of Health, London.

DoH (2000d) *Folic Acid and the Prevention of Disease*. Report on Health and Social Subjects 50. The Stationery Office, London.

Gregory, J. *et al.* (2000) *National Diet and Nutrition Survey: young people aged 4-18 years. 1: Findings*. The Stationery Office, London.

HDA (2000) *Prevention of Coronary Heart Disease through Promoting Healthier Lifestyles*. Health Development Agency, London.

Hillsden, M., Thorogood, M. & Foster, C. (1999) A systematic review of strategies to promote physical activity. In: *Benefits and Hazards of Exercise*, vol. 1 (ed. D. MacAuley), pp. 25-46, British Medical Association, London.

MAG (2000) *Guidelines for Detection and Management of Malnutrition*. Malnutrition Advisory Group, London.

Maryon Davis, A., Giles, A. & Rona, R. (2000) *Tackling Obesity: a toolbox for local partnership action*. Faculty of Public Health of the Royal College of Physicians, London.

Petersen, S., Mockford, C. & Rayner, M. (1999) *Coronary Heart Disease Statistics: 1999 edition*. British Heart Foundation, London.

Prentice, A.M. & Jebb, S.A. (1995) Obesity in Britain: gluttony or sloth? *BMJ*, **311**, 437-9.

CLOSING SPEECH TO CONFERENCE

SUZI LEATHER

Thank you very much for inviting me to give the closing speech for this important conference and it is great to see the re-emergence of interest in nutrition on the part of health professionals. With so many conflicting demands on your time during your training and now your work for the Health Service, it is sometimes hard to remember the vital contribution of nutrition to health throughout the whole of life, including in the womb. Historically health improvement and public health with the NHS have had a low status, and within public health, food and nutrition have received less attention. Now we recognise that nutrition has a vital part to play in achieving the government's health targets for cardiovascular disease and cancer, but we also recognise that there are other factors such as income and education which are important determinants of health.

Positive moves in the past have included adding an element of nutrition education into the medical curriculum, and increasingly the professional colleges have been taking an interest in nutrition, particularly from the point of view of prevention. But we know that a patient's nutritional status may barely register as a blip on the radar of the average GP as he or she rushes through a series of five or ten minute consultations. It is time to spread the message more widely, and this conference has provided a comprehensive state of the art review of the latest knowledge in all areas of nutrition.

As you know, until recently government responsibility for food lay with the Ministry of Agriculture, Fisheries and Food (MAFF). While MAFF continues to have responsibility for food production, the Food Standards Agency has taken over responsibility for food safety issues and nutrition since April 2000. Safety has been the dominant concern in food debate most recently, indeed it was the BSE scandal which led to the setting up of the Food Standards Agency. But, put in perspective, mortality from problems associated with nutrition far outstrips that from food poisoning. The complexity comes from the fact that chronic diseases are multi-factorial in origin and the contribution that improved nutrition can make may vary a great deal depending on the disease. In addition to which, we still do not fully understand the true role of some foods or components of foods in preventing degenerative conditions.

The Food Standards Agency has very specific responsibilities in relation to nutrition, which include collecting and communicating up-to-date information on food composition, and providing a definition of a balanced diet for use in health education material. We can provide practical guidance in relation to nutritional aspects of the food chain from farm to fork.

The Food Standards Agency funds jointly with the Department of Health the National Diet and Nutrition Surveys. The Survey of Young People was published in June 2000, and provides an extraordinarily detailed and revealing portrait of the dietary habits and nutritional status of the participants, who were aged between 4 and 18 years. We are extremely grateful to these young people for making the commitment to collect full 7 day weighed records and provide their body measurements, blood and urine samples. The findings highlighted that there are significant numbers of young people with low fruit and vegetable intake – during the survey week more than half of young people had not eaten any citrus fruits or leafy green vegetables. Physical activity levels fell with age, and teenage girls turned out to be the real couch potatoes which is a particular concern since 36% of girls also reported smoking and we know that both of these factors predispose to osteoporosis later in life.

The surveys provide us with data on socio-demographic factors which can militate against the taking up of the healthy eating messages which we know so well, but which are often inaccessible, particularly to those with the worst health and life chances. Food choice is not just determined by education or knowledge but also social class, income and access. We found that children from low income families had a different pattern of food consumption, and in particular were less likely to consume raw and salad vegetables, fruit juice and soft fruits. On the other hand, they were less likely to eat cream and butter. We found that vitamin C levels in the blood increased with income, and although deficiency by the standard definition was rare, it may well be that this is still not satisfactory since we are beginning to realise that to prevent degenerative diseases, higher intakes of nutrients such as vitamin C are needed than those normally required just to prevent classic deficiency diseases.

The Food Standards Agency also funds several nutrition research programmes inherited from the Ministry of Agriculture, Fisheries and Food. Through the funding of research the Agency will continue to contribute to the growing body of knowledge on, for example, components of fruits and vegetables which may contribute to disease prevention. We will also be looking at developing new methods for assessing the diets of those on low incomes, with a view to a new diet and nutrition survey of low income families. Some new research will also flow from the work of the new Scientific Advisory Committee on Nutrition which is now being set up jointly by the Food Standards Agency and the Department of Health.

The Food Standards Agency is committed to working closely with government bodies which are also involved with nutrition, including the Department of Health, the Department for Education and Employment, and the Health Development Agency.

Staff of the Food Standards Agency also work closely with non-governmental organisations such as the British Nutrition Foundation. Through the funding of research under the Food Acceptability and Choice programme we are concerned with exploring, for example, ways in which we might intervene with youngsters to prevent obesity developing later in life, discovering whether the concept of food deserts is genuine and looking at ways to encourage people to develop and enjoy cookery skills. Good nutrition is about much more than knowing your vitamins and minerals.

The point now, as the title of this section of the conference (From research to practice: implementation) suggests, is how do we move from the realm of the laboratory to the real world. The public are bombarded with a huge diversity of information about food and nutrition, some of which is questionable. Sometimes healthy eating messages have been perceived as confusing or too difficult to put into practice. This is a sensitive area since healthy eating messages from government compete with concern about the 'nanny state' curbing individual choice, and commercial interests of food and drink manufacturers. The benefits of dietary change are not immediate in our 'instant' society.

So what is the role of the health sector? Let's take General Practice. Recent bad publicity has no doubt made the profession feel beleaguered, but let's remind ourselves of the strengths of the primary care team. There is no doubt that General Practice is still a source of respected advice for the general public; 75% of the population see their GP in any given year, and 95% over a five year period. Members of the primary care team provide one-to-one contact and an opportunity for giving preventive advice which is personalised. General Practitioners still have the unique strength of being able to get to know not just the individual but often the entire family over two or three generations, although this is more difficult where populations are more mobile.

The primary care team also includes community health professionals of all kinds, including the health visitor, community midwife, dietitians, school nurses, community dentists, pharmacists and many others, all of whom have the chance to get to know people and have the advantage of understanding local conditions and the factors that will help individuals make the best choices in order to lead healthy lives. All of these professionals see people at times in their lives when they may well be open to change, for example during pregnancy, when women are otherwise normally healthy but for the first time in some instances are focused on what is best for their unborn child which is often, as it happens, best for the mother as well.

On the down side, many people do not think about change until it is too late, when they are ill, and the medical setting may provide only damage limitation. But in some cases, better late than never, and substantial improvements in life expectancy and quality of life can be gained by secondary prevention after a heart attack or stroke, although we know that this may mean a multi-pronged approach using drugs as well as healthy living advice such as increasing exercise and improving diet.

As a health professional, whether based in hospital or in the community, you can never assume that your client or patient is adequately fed or has the means to provide an adequate diet for themselves or their children. It is a sad fact that one in three children in Britain lives in poverty, that is to say, they live in households whose income is less than half average earnings. Many of these live in lone parent households, the majority of whom are on Income Support. The consequences of this are enormous, at the same time physical, mental and social, from poor iron status in infancy leading to slower development, to social stigma from being different to others.

With recent advances in the Health Service, nutrition is being kept on the agenda via Health Improvement Programmes. Government initiatives such as Sure Start and the New Children's Fund for school age children have already been addressing some of the problems associated with poverty in childhood. There is no doubt that newly established Primary Care Groups and Trusts will also have an interest in prevention through their key role in population health development.

The new NHS Plan has also identified nutrition as a key factor in reducing ill health, in conjunction with improved health services. This will involve, for example, joint working between the Food Standards Agency and the Department of Health to work towards reducing the salt content of manufactured foods. This is a population-based approach which primary care professionals would not be able to address since 75% of the salt we consume is already added to pre-prepared foods and consumers would not be able to avoid this with simple healthy eating advice. This illustrates well how no single approach can solve the problems we are addressing.

I believe that the time is right to give diet further prominence in our work. As an organisation the Food Standards Agency will be working closely with others to improve the evidence base for targeted research and effective interventions, for example by working with the Health Development Agency. We can work towards improving food labelling, and giving clearer advice to consumers. In Scotland and Wales the Food Standards Agency is working closely with their Parliament and Assembly to bring improvements to areas of the UK with particularly marked problems such as the highest rates of coronary heart disease in the world.

We need to think about developing guidance on models for local dietary improvement, perhaps by looking at best practice in community involvement and consultation, and evaluating diet and nutrition goals at HImP level. Health Improvement Programmes provide a start from which local partnerships can be identified and strengthened to deliver local and hence national targets. We will continue to look at the population-based approaches which will complement your own work with individuals, because after all that is what it all boils down to: the patient or client sitting in your surgery or in their own home. Don't underestimate the power of a single consultation: we know that a few minutes with a GP can persuade someone to stop smoking; there is certainly potential to influence people at an individual level given the right approaches. Together we can take on this responsibility with enthusiasm.

It remains for me to thank the organisers once again for inviting me to close this excellent conference, and I hope that you have all found it a fruitful event, so to speak!

Appendices:

WORKSHOPS HELD DURING THE FIRST NUTRITION AND HEALTH CONFERENCE

LC-PUFAS: THEIR ROLE IN MATERNAL AND INFANT NUTRITION

STEWART FORSYTH

LC-PUFAs and infant cognitive development

Several observational studies have indicated that breast fed children are intellectually advantaged compared to children who were formula fed. However, it is recognised that these studies involved non-random assignment to groups and other factors such as genetic and social-demographic variables, parenting skills, or quality of parent-child inter-action which may also contribute to differences in cognitive abilities. Attempts to statistically control for the potentially confounding effects of these factors may be inadequate (Wright & Deary, 1992). The role of LC-PUFAs in cognitive development can be studied by randomising infants to formulas containing either LC-PUFAs or no LC-PUFAs. Randomised studies of the effects of LC-PUFAs on development in both term and preterm infants have employed a variety of assessments, which include tests of psychomotor development, language development, visual attention, and problem solving.

LC-PUFAs and infant psychomotor and language development

Standardised tests such as the Bayley Scales (Bayley, 1993) provide global measures of infant psychomotor development. Carlson (1994) rando-mised preterm infants to formula containing either no LC-PUFAs or a supplement containing both EPA and DHA. Bayley Mental Developmental

Index (MDI) scores at corrected age 12 months did not differ between the groups, but Psychomotor Developmental Index (PDI) scores tended to be lower in the EPA + DHA supplemented group, a result that was consistent with the finding of poorer growth in preterm infants supplemented with DHA and relatively high levels of EPA (Carlson *et al.*, 1992). In a second study in which the DHA content of the supplemented formula remained the same but the EPA content was reduced, Carlson (1994) reported significantly higher MDI scores in preterm infants aged 12 months who received n-3 LC-PUFAs in comparison to the control group. Damli *et al.* (1996) also reported higher MDI scores in 6-month-old preterm infants who were fed formula supplemented with AA + DHA in comparison to infants receiving no supplement.

Two randomised studies have examined the effects of LC-PUFA supplementation on measures of psychomotor development in term infants. Agostoni *et al.* (1995) compared scores on the Brunet-Lézine test in two groups of infants fed a formula containing no LC-PUFAs or supplemented with AA + DHA. Significantly higher test scores were observed in the LC-PUFA-supplemented group at age 4 months, but no differences were found in a follow up conducted at age 24 months (Agostoni *et al.*, 1997). In a multi-centre study reported by Scott *et al.*, (1997), scores on the Bayley Scales were compared in three groups of infants at age 12 months. The groups received either standard formula containing no LC-PUFAs, formula containing DHA, or formula containing AA and DHA. No differences were observed in either MDI or PDI scores. Lucas and colleagues (1999) randomised 309 infants from four hospitals to formulas with or without DHA and AA. At age 18 months Bayley's MDI scores did not differ between the two randomised groups. In contrast, Birch and colleagues (2000) showed in a smaller cohort that infants supplemented with both DHA and AA had a seven point advantage compared to unsupplemented infants.

Although there is considerable evidence to suggest that preformed dietary LC-PUFAs enhance the rate of infant psychomotor development during the first year of life, particularly in preterm infants, there is a lack of consistency in the results. This may be related to the items on the Bayley Mental Scale which are employed in children younger than 2 years tending to measure perceptual-motor abilities rather than important cognitive changes that may predict later intellectual ability (Roberts *et al.*, 1999). This is supported by data showing that scores achieved on standardised tests of infant development correlate poorly with later measures of childhood intelligence (Slater, 1995). For these reasons, researchers have employed other assessments to identify more specific effects of LC-PUFAs on infant cognitive function.

Infant visual information processing

Habituation is an inhibitory process involving a decline in attention paid to a stimulus. Behaviourally, visual habituation is the decrease in looking time that occurs when a stimulus becomes familiar (Ruff & Rothbart, 1996). Infant habituation involves active processing of information and memory for a stimulus. Recognition of the familiar (habituated) stimulus is demonstrated by longer looking at a novel stimulus compared to the familiar stimulus in a paired-comparison test involving presentation of both stimuli for a fixed duration (Bornstein, 1985; Colombo, 1993; Slater, 1995). Look duration shows modest but significant correlations with childhood cognitive measures such as IQ and vocabulary scores (Colombo, 1993; McCall & Carriger, 1993; Slater, 1995). These correlations are negative, with children who demonstrated more efficient habituation (shorter total looking times and shorter individual look durations) having higher IQ and vocabulary scores.

An alternative to habituation for investigating infant visual information processing and memory is the visual recognition memory (VRM) paradigm (Colombo, 1993; Slater 1995). In the VRM paradigm, infants are initially familiarised to either a single stimulus or pair of identical stimuli for a fixed and relatively short duration. Infants subsequently receive a paired-comparison test in which the proportion of looking time directed at the novel stimulus (novelty-preference score) indicates the extent to which information about the familiarised stimulus was processed and encoded in memory.

LC-PUFAs and infant visual information processing

Only one study has examined the relationship between LC-PUFA supplementation and infant habituation (Forsyth & Willatts, 1996). Term infants were randomised to formulas containing AA + DHA or no LC-PUFAs, and measures of visual habituation were obtained at age 3 months. Although LC-PUFA-supplemented infants tended to have shorter fixation durations, none of the overall comparisons between the groups was significant. However, infants who had late peak fixations and who may have been more distractible had significantly shorter total fixation durations if they received LC-PUFA supplementation in comparison to infants who received no LC-PUFAs. Infants with late peak fixations also had reduced growth parameters at birth compared to infants with early peak fixations. Duration of fixation in infants with early peak fixations was not influenced by LC-PUFA supplementation. These results suggest that infants who have suffered moderate intra-uterine undernutrition may develop more efficient information processing if they are supplemented with LC-PUFAs.

Three randomised studies have examined the relationship between LC-PUFA supplementation and performance on the Fagan Test of Infant Intelligence. Clausen *et al.* (1996) reported significantly higher novelty-preference scores in term infants fed a formula supplemented with AA + DHA compared to infants fed a formula containing no LC-PUFAs. In two studies of preterm infants (Carlson & Werkman, 1996; Werkman & Carlson, 1996), infants received formula containing either no LC-PUFAs or DHA + EPA which had a relatively high ratio of DHA to EPA. No significant differences between the diet groups were found on novelty-preference scores, but fixation durations in paired-comparison tests were shorter in the supplemented groups. In the study by Carlson and Werkman (1996), LC-PUFA supplementation was stopped at age 2 months but the effects on look duration were seen at age 12 months.

The consistency of these findings suggests that preformed dietary LC-PUFAs (and in particular, n-3 LC-PUFAs) are important for more efficient infant visual information processing. These effects do not appear to be related to the reported effects of LC-PUFAs on visual acuity development (e.g. Makrides *et al.*, 1995; Birch *et al.*, 1998) because look duration and acuity scores are not correlated (Carlson *et al.*, 1995; Neuringer *et al.*, 1996; Jacobson, 1999).

Infant means-end problem solving

Means-end problem solving involves the deliberate and planned execution of a sequence of steps to achieve a goal, and this ability develops rapidly after 6 months of age (Willatts, 1989). Infants aged between 7 and 8 months begin to solve simple one-step problems such as searching under a cover for a toy, or pulling a cloth to retrieve a toy that is resting on it (Willatts, 1984, 1999). At 9 months, infants can solve more complex problems requiring the completion of two intermediate steps to achieve a goal (Willatts, 1997). Two-step problem-solving scores measured at 9 months correlate positively with IQ and vocabulary scores measured at 3 years (Slater, 1995; Willatts, 1997). Infants at 10 months can solve more complex problems which require the execution of three intermediate steps to achieve a goal (Willatts & Rosie, 1992). It is not known whether ability at three-step problem solving is related to childhood cognitive scores.

Means-end problem solving involves planning, sequencing actions, and maintaining attention to a goal, all of which are mediated by prefrontal cortex (Diamond, 1991; Johnson, 1997; Roberts *et al.*, 1998). There is some evidence linking infants' ability at means-end problem solving to development of prefrontal cortex (Bell & Fox, 1992; Diamond *et al.*, 1997), but a direct link between performance on multi-step means-end problems and prefrontal cortex has yet to be established.

LC-PUFAs and infant problem solving

Infants who were randomised to a formula, with or without DHA and AA, were assessed at the age of 10 months (Willatts *et al.*, 1998). They were given a task to complete three intermediate steps to achieve a final goal and solve the problem (remove a barrier to grasp a cloth, pull the cloth to retrieve a cover, and search under the cover to find a hidden toy). Infants who received the LC-PUFA-supplemented formula had significantly higher problem-solving scores than infants who received no LC-PUFAs.

These results suggest that problem solving is improved in term infants who received formula supplemented with LC-PUFAs, and the benefits of LC-PUFA supplementation to infants persist beyond the period that they received their supplemented formula. The differences between the diet groups may reflect faster information processing and therefore more efficient problem solving in the LC-PUFA-supplemented group. Alternatively, they may reflect improved ability at disengagement in the LC-PUFA-supplemented group. Infants who can easily disengage attention from a stimulus may be able to switch rapidly from manipulating one intermediary to the next, and so solve a complex means-end problem.

Conclusions

Although the number of studies of the effects of preformed dietary LC-PUFAs on infant cognitive function is relatively small, a consistent pattern of findings is beginning to emerge. In the majority of studies, both term and preterm infants fed artificial formula supplemented with LC-PUFAs (DHA or AA + DHA) showed improved cognitive performance in comparison to control infants fed a formula containing no LC-PUFAs. No negative effects on development have been observed with formulas containing both AA and DHA. Only two studies have reported poorer cognitive scores in groups receiving LC-PUFA supplement (Carlson, 1994; Scott *et al.*, 1997). These studies share two features that may be related to these effects. First, the supplement was DHA without AA. Second, the DHA source was marine oil that also included EPA. This suggests that the ratios of EPA to DHA and AA to DHA are more relevant to cognitive outcome than the absolute level of DHA. This conclusion is reinforced by the fact that in studies reporting a significant cognitive advantage in infants who received LC-PUFA supplement, formulas were supplemented with AA + DHA or DHA with low EPA.

References

Agostoni, C., Trojan, S., Bellù R., Riva, E. & Giovannini, M. (1995) Neurodevelopmental quotient of healthy term infants at 4 months and feeding practice: The role of long chain polyunsaturated fatty acids. *Pediatr. Res.*, **38**, 262–6.

Agostoni, C., Trojan, S., Bellù, R., Riva, E., Bruzzese, M.G. & Giovannini, M. (1997) Developmental quotient at 24 months and fatty acid composition of diet in early infancy: A follow up study. *Archiv. Dis. Child.*, **76**, 421–4.

Bayley, N. (1993) *The Bayley Scales of Infant Development*, 2nd edn. The Psychological Corporation, San Antonio.

Bell, M.A. & Fox, N. (1992) The relations between frontal brain electrical activity and cognitive development during infancy. *Child Dev.*, **63**, 1142–63.

Birch, E.B. Hoffman, D.R. Uauy, R. Birch, D.G. & Prestidge, C. (1998) Visual acuity and the essentiality of docosahexaenoic acid and arachidonic acid in the diet of term infants. *Pediatr. Res.*, **44**, 201–9.

Birch, E.B., Garfield, S., Hoffman, D.R. & Uauy, R. (2000) A randomised controlled trial of early dietary supply of long-chain polyunsaturated fatty acids and mental development in term infants. *Dev. Med. Child. Neur.*, **42**, 174–81.

Bornstein, M.H. (1985) Habituation of attention as a measure of visual information processing in human infants: Summary, systematization, and synthesis. In: *Measurement of Audition and Vision in the First Year of Postnatal Life: A methodological overview* (eds G. Gottlieb & N.A. Krasnegor), pp. 253–300. Ablex, Norwood.

Carlson, S.E. (1994) Growth and development of premature infants in relation to n3 and n6 fatty status. In: *Fatty Acids and Lipids: Biological aspects* (eds C. Gali, A.P. Simopolous, & E. Tremoli). Karger, Basel: 63–9.

Carlson, S.E. & Werkman, S.H. (1996) A randomised trial of visual attention of preterm infants fed docosahexaenoic acid until two months. *Lipids*, **31**, 85–90.

Carlson, S.E., Werkman, S.H. & Peeples, J.M. (1995) Early visual acuity does not correlate with later evidence of visual processing in preterm infants although each is improved by the addition of docosahexaenoic acid to infants formula. *Abstract in Second International Congress of the International Society for the Study of Fatty Acids (ISSFAL)*, p. 53. American Oil Chemist's Society, Champaign.

Carlson, S.E. Rhodes, P.G. & Ferguson, M.G. (1992) First year growth of preterm infants fed standard compared to marine oil n-3 supplemented formula. *Lipids*, **27**, 901–7.

Clausen, U., Damli, A., von Schenck, U. & Koletzko, B. (1996) Influence of long-chain polyunsaturated fatty acids (LC-PUFAs) on early visual acuity and mental development of term infants. *Abstracts of the AOCS Conference, PUFA in Infant Nutrition: Consensus and Controversies*, p. 12. American Oil Chemist's Society, Champaign.

Colombo, J. (1993) *Infant Cognition: Predicting Later Intellectual Functioning*. Sage, London.

Damli, A., von Schenck, U., Clausen, U. & Koletzko, B. (1996) Effects of long-chain polyunsaturated fatty acids (LC-PUFAs) on early visual acuity and mental development in preterm infants. *Abstracts of the AOCS Conference, PUFA in Infant Nutrition: Consensus and Controversies*, p. 14. American Oil Chemist's Society, Champaign.

Diamond, A. (1991) Neuropsychological insights into the meaning of object concept development. In: *The Epigenesis of Mind: Essays on biology and cognition*, (eds S. Carey & R. Gelman), pp. 67–110. Erlbaum, Hillsdale.

Diamond, A., Prevor, M.B., Callender, G. & Druin, D.P. (1997) Prefrontal cortex deficits in children treated early and continuously for PKU. *Monogr. Soc. Res. Child Dev.*, Serial No. 252, 62, Whole no. 4.

Forsyth, J.S. & Willatts, P. (1996) Do LC-PUFAs influence infant cognitive behavior? In: *Recent Developments in Infant Nutrition* (eds J.G. Bindels, A.C. Goedhart, & H.K.A. Visser), pp. 225–34. Kluwer Academic, Dordrecht.

Jacobson, S.W. (1999) Assessment of long-chain polyunsaturated fatty acid nutritional supplementation on infant neurobehavioral development and visual acuity. *Lipids*, 34, 151–60.

Johnson, M.H. (1997) *Developmental Cognitive Neuroscience*. Blackwell, Oxford.

Lucas, A., Stafford, M., Morley, R., Abbott, R., Stephenson, T., MacFadyen, U., Elias-Jones, A. & Clements, H. (1999) Efficacy and safety of long-chain polyunsaturated fatty acid supplementation of infant-formula milk: a randomised trial. *Lancet*, 354, 1948–54.

Makrides, M., Neumann, M., Simmer, K., Pater, J. & Gibson, R.A. (1995) Are long-chain polyunsaturated fatty acids essential nutrients in infancy? *Lancet*, 345, 1463–68.

McCall, R.B. & Carriger, M.S. (1993) A meta-analysis of infant habituation and recognition memory performance as predictors of later IQ. *Child Dev.*, 64, 57–79.

Neuringer, M., Reisbick, S. & Teemer, C. (1996) Relationships between visual acuity and visual attention measures in rhesus monkey infants. *Invest., Ophthalmol. Vis. Sci.*, 37, S532.

Roberts, A.C., Robbins, T.W. & Weiskrantz, L. (1998) *The prefrontal cortex: Executive and cognitive functions*. Oxford University Press, Oxford.

Roberts, E., Bornstein, M.H., Slater, A. & Barrett, J. (1999) Early cognitive development and parental education. *Infant Child Dev.*, 8, 49–62.

Ruff, H.A. & Rothbart, M.K. (1996) *Attention in Early Development: Themes and variations*. Oxford University Press, Oxford.

Scott, D.T., Janowsky, J.S., Hall, R.T.,Wheeler, R.E., Jacobsen, C.H., Auestad, N. & Monalto, M.B. (1997) Cognitive and language assessment of 3.25 yr old children fed formula with or without long chain polyunsaturated fatty acids (LCP) in the first year of life. *Pediatr. Res.*, 41, 240A.

Slater, A. (1995) Individual differences in infancy and later IQ. *J. Child Psychol. Psychiatr.*, **36**, 69–112.

Werkman, S.H. & Carlson, S.E. (1996) A randomized trial of usual attention of preterm infants fed docosahexaenoic acid until nine months. *Lipids*, **31**, 97–7.

Willatts, P. (1984) Stages in the development of intentional search by young infants. *Dev. Psych.*, **20**, 389–96.

Willatts, P. (1989) Development of problem solving in infancy. In: *Infant development* (eds A. Slater & J.G. Bremner), pp. 143–82. Erlbaum, London.

Willatts, P. (1997) Beyond the 'couch potato' infant: How infants use their knowledge to regulate action, solve problems, and achieve goals. In: *Infant Development: Recent Advances* (eds J.G. Bremner, A. Slater & G. Butterworth), pp. 109–35. Psychology Press, Hove.

Willatts, P. (1999) Development of means-end behavior in young infants: Pulling a support to retrieve a distant object. *Dev. Psych.*, **35**, 651–67.

Willatts, P., Forsyth, J.S., DiModugno, M.K., Varma, S. & Colvin, M. (1998) Effect of long-chain polyunsaturated fatty acids in infant formula on problem solving at 10 months of age. *Lancet*, **352**, 688–91.

Willatts, P. & Rosie, K. (1992) Thinking ahead: Development of means-end planning in young infants. *Infant Beh. Dev.*, **15**, 769.

Wright, P. & Deary, I.J. (1992) Breastfeeding and intelligence. *Lancet*, **339**, 612.

SOYA IN WOMEN'S HEALTH

PAOLA ALBERTAZZI

Introduction

Epidemiological data suggest that Asian women have a lower incidence of hot flushes compared to Western women as well as a lower incidence of coronary artery disease and estrogen dependent cancers such as that of the breast. Soy is a staple ingredient of the traditional oriental diet and contains large quantities of phytoestrogens. These compounds have an oestrogen-like structure and their use has been proposed in the treatment of post-menopausal women. Women with contra-indications to the use of conventional oestrogen replacement, or simply wanting a more 'natural' alternative to relieve their distressing menopausal symptoms are increasingly requesting information about the efficacy of these forms of diet supplementation.

Several clinical trials on vasomotor symptoms have been performed to date using various forms of phytoestrogen supplementation, sometimes with contradictory results. Two very preliminary studies seem to suggest a beneficial effect of diet supplemented with soy for the prevention of post-menopausal bone loss. Prospective long-term human data are still lacking on the effect of soy supplementation on breast and endometrium.

This chapter will critically review the clinical data available to date in an attempt to answer some of the most commonly asked questions about dose and type of phytoestrogen supplementation most likely to be effective for climacteric symptom relief. Phytoestrogens are plant-derived molecules so named because they possess oestrogen-like activity.

Soy has been a staple in the diet of the populations in the Far East for centuries. Its consumption has been related to high longevity rates together with a low incidence of breast cancer (Parkin *et al.*, 1993) and dementia (Ichinowatari *et al.*, 1987; Graves *et al.*, 1996) in this population. Soy is unique among foods in that it contains large amounts of isoflavones, a group of polyphenols thought to be active components of soy. Isoflavones can stimulate the transcriptional activity of oestrogen receptors (ER) particularly ERβ (Kuiper *et al.*, 1998). For this reason they are often called phytoestrogens, although they also have several other biological and antioxidant properties. Japanese women consuming a traditional diet have been found to have a low incidence of breast cancer, cardiovascular disease, osteoporosis and climacteric symptoms whilst the men have a very low incidence of prostate cancer. The high concentration of soy-derived isoflavones present in their diet has been adduced to explain these findings at least partially. Whether increasing phytoestrogens in the diet of Western men and women would have a favourable influence on health is currently unresolved and is receiving much attention. But if it is proven, phytoestrogen might be an ideal alternative to steroid hormones, as it might have both a bone sparing, and an athero protective effect without any negative influence on the reproductive system.

Climacteric symptoms

There have been eleven randomised studies on incidence and severity of hot flushes in peri and post-menopausal women. Five studies have used whole grain or soy preparation containing proteins (Murkies *et al.*, 1995; Brzezinski *et al.*, 1997; Dalais *et al.*, 1998; Albertazzi *et al.*, 1998; Washburn *et al.*, 1999) while five studies have used concentrated isoflavones in tablet form either derived from soy (Quella *et al.*, 2000; Scambia *et al.*, 2000; Upmalis *et al.*, 2000) or red clover (Knight *et al.*, 1999; Baber *et al.*, 1999). All the studies performed with phytoestrogen were randomised, nine were double-blind and all but two had a placebo arm.

Albertazzi *et al.* showed that 60 g of isolated soy protein powder containing 40 g of proteins and 76 mg phytoestrogens, in the aglycone active form, has been shown to halve the number of hot flushes in post-menopausal women in a double-blind, placebo controlled trial. During this study a coincidental brief decrease in the daily amount of powder intake was mirrored by a marked reduction in efficacy. Sixty grams of isolated soy protein powder containing 76 mg of phytoestrogens appear, thus, to be the minimal effective dose required for reduction of vasomotor symptoms in post-menopausal women. In this study, soy did not have any effects on the important oestrogen-sensitive symptom of vaginal dryness.

Brzezinski *et al.*, compared a diet high in phytoestrogen with one containing low phytoestrogen on hot flushes in post-menopausal women. The phytoestrogen rich diet consisted of a daily consumption of 80 g/day tofu (75 mg/g daidzeine, 200 mg/g genistein), 400 ml of soy drink (7 mg/g daidzeine, 20 mg/g genistein), 1 teaspoon of miso (40 mg/g daidzein, 35 mg/g genistein), 2 teaspoons of ground linseeds (4 mg/g lignans). This would amount to a consumption of approximately 33 mg of phytoestrogens per day. This was found to be effective in reducing hot flushes and improving vaginal dryness. This study, however, was not double-blind, something difficult to achieve when using conventional food, but important to consider when interpreting results since hot flushes exhibit a high placebo response.

Murkies *et al.* in a double-blind, non-placebo-controlled study, found a 40% reduction in the number of hot flushes using 45 g of soy flour per day (approximately 23–90 mg of phytoestrogens) but a similar amount of wheat flour used as control also reduced hot flushes by about 20%.

Dalais *et al.* (1998) carried out a crossover study using high phytoestrogen-containing foods – 45 g of soy grit, 45 g of linseeds – versus a low phytoestrogen-containing food – 45 g of wheat kibble turned into bread. The study involved a total of 52 women but only 44 completed the study. In this study the soy bread did not affect hot flushes but significantly improved the maturation of the vaginal epithelium. Hot flushes were significantly reduced by the wheat and the linseed bread. Admittedly, the sample size was rather small, and the study had only a 60% power to detect a decrease of 40% in hot flushes.

Washburn *et al.* observed a reduction in only the severity of hot flushes but not in their number by supplementing the diet of 51 peri-menopausal women with 20 g of soy protein containing 34 mg of phytoestrogen. The less than impressive results might have been due, at least partially, to the study design itself. The eligibility criteria allowed participation to women who had missed as few as three menstrual periods in the preceding 12 months. It is standard practice to allow participation in trials of this kind only to women with at least 6 months of amenorrhoea in order to minimise chances of improvement in symptoms due to sporadic production of endogenous oestrogen. Furthermore, women taking part in this trial had as little as one hot flush per day or night. Given the levity of the starting symptoms, a much larger sample size might have been necessary to observe a small effect with treatment.

Kotsopoulus *et al.* (2000) found no climacteric symptom relief in 94 post-menopausal women enrolled in a three months double-blind, placebo trial using soy supplements containing 118 mg of isoflavones per day. The study design had, however, several limitations. Women were not required to keep a daily account of the number of hot flushes, but symptoms were scored only in terms of climacteric questionnaires: a less accurate estimation of symptom intensity. Furthermore, women enrolled in this study had only mild climacteric symptoms; this might have also contributed to the underestimation of all but a major effect of the treatment under trial.

Two studies have been performed with concentrated phytoestrogens tablets derived from red clover. In these studies doses of 40 and 160 mg failed to reduce hot flushes over a 3 month period (Baber *et al.*, 1999; Knight *et al.*, 1999). These studies both involved only a small number of women and, once again, the small sample size might have unfavourably influenced outcome.

Two randomised placebo-controlled studies have been performed with tablets containing isoflavones derived from soy. Each of the tablets contained 50 mg of phytoestrogens and a decrease of between 28 and 45% in the number of hot flushes was observed (Scambia *et al.*, 2000; Upmalis *et al.*, 2000). On the other hand, Quella *et al.* did not show any reduction in hot flushes in breast cancer survivors using 150 mg of phytoestrogen in tablets (Quella *et al.*, 2000). This study, again, had several flaws. The cross-over design had two phases lasting only 4 weeks which were not separated by a wash out period. Thus a carry-over effect cannot be excluded. The number of patients studied was substantial, 177, but over half of them had a minor symptomatology (17% with 2–3 hot flushes per day and 50% with 4–9 hot flushes per day). Furthermore, 70% of women on the trial were taking tamoxifen and it might thus be speculated that a larger dose of phytoestrogen might have been required to overcome the known anti-oestrogenic action of tamoxifen on the central nervous system. Lastly, the authors did not specify the quantity of isoflavones, if any, that were present in the aglycone form in the tablets. Low levels of isoflavones in the aglycone-active form might have affected the overall efficacy of treatment.

Vaginal dryness is a frequent complaint in post-menopausal women. It is usually assessed either in term of intensity of symptoms or, more objectively, by cytological assessment of maturation of vaginal epithelium. Eight studies have looked at maturation of vaginal epithelium (Wilcox *et al.*, 1990; Baird *et al.*, 1995; Murkies *et al.*, 1995; Albertazzi *et al.*, 1998; Dalais *et al.*, 1998; Baber *et al.*, 1999; Knight *et al.*, 1999; Upmalis *et al.*, 2000) with phytoestrogen supplementation. Two studies (Wilcox *et al.*, 1990; Dalais *et al.*, 1998) found it to be improved, but one of these studies was of only 2 weeks duration (Wilcox *et al.*, 1990). No changes were observed in vaginal maturation in the remaining six studies.

Endocrinological effect

Do phytoestrogens have an effect on the thyroid gland? *In vitro* studies have suggested that isolated isoflavones may inhibit thyroid peroxidase (Divi & Doerge, 1996; Divi *et al.*, 1997), but these data have not been confirmed in animal studies (Chang & Doerge, 2000). Furthermore, no thyroid function abnormalities have been found in either pre-menopausal (Duncan *et al.*, 1999a) or post-menopausal (Duncan *et al.*, 1999b) women fed soy powder containing up to 132 mg of isoflavones, while a reduction has been shown in insulin levels. This latter finding might suggest a possible favourable effect of soy supplementation in the prevention or type 2 diabetes.

Effect of phytoestrogen on cognitive function

A lower incidence of dementia is found in Asian populations particularly amongst Japanese (Graves *et al.*, 1996). Prospective human data is lacking but ovariectomised rats fed with a soy preparation rich in phytoestrogen had an improvement in radial arm maze performance comparable to that of oestrogen. The radial maze performance is an expression of working memory, and the beneficial effect obtained with soy was dose-related and did not antagonise the effects of oestrogen when the two compounds were given together (Pan *et al.*, 2000).

Effect on the bone

There have been several *in vitro* and animal studies that have shown that dietary soybean prevents bone loss (Arjmandi *et al.*, 1996), but to date only two human studies have been reported. Forty mg of isolated soy protein containing 90 mg of isoflavones determined a 2.2% increase in the lumbar spine bone mineral density compared with baseline. This difference was statistically significant (Potter *et al.*, 1998). The study was double-blind and placebo-controlled involving 66 post-menopausal women but only lasted 6 months. The second similar study was performed in 69 peri-menopausal/menopausal women. Eighty mg of phytoestrogen in the daily diet prevented lumbar spine bone loss while 1.28% loss was observed in the placebo group (Alekel *et al.*, 2000).

Conclusions

Supplementing the western diet with phytoestrogen-containing food does appear to mildly reduce hot flushes and might have a bone sparing effect without adverse effects on breast and endometrium. All the studies performed so far have, however, been very short. Further longer term data are now needed.

References

Albertazzi, P., Pansini, F., Bonaccorsi, G., Zanotti, L., Forini, E. & De Aloysio, D. (1998) The effects of soy supplementation on hot flushes. *Obstet. Gynecol.*, **91**, 6–11.

Alekel, D.L., Germain, A.S., Peterson, C.T., Hanson, K.B., Steward, J.W. & Toda, T. (2000) Isoflavone-rich soy protein isolate attenuate bone loss in the lumbar spine of perimanopausal women. *Am. J. Clin. Nutr.*, **72**, 844–52.

Arjmandi, B.H., Alekel, L., Hollis, B.W., Amin, D., Stacewicz-Sapuntzakis, M., Guo, P. & Kukreja, S.C. (1996) Dietary soybean prevents bone loss in an ovariectomised rat model of osteoporosis. *J. Nutr.*, **126**, 161–7.

Baber, R.J., Templeman, C., Morton, T., Kelly, G.E.& West, L. (1999) Randomised placebo-controlled trial of an isoflavone supplement and menopausal symptom in women. *Climcacteric*, **2**, 85–92.

Baird, D.D., Umbach, D.M., Lansdell, L. *et al.* (1995) Dietary intervention study to assess estrogenincity of dietary soy amongst postmenopausal women. *J. Clin. Endocrin Metab.*, **80**, 1685–90.

Brzezinski, A., Adlercreutz, H, Shaoul, R., Rosler, A., Shmueli, A., Tanos, V. & Schenker, G.J. (1997) Short-term effects of phytoestrogen-rich diet on postmenopausal women. *Menopause*, **4**, 89–94.

Chang, H.C. & Doerge, D.R. (2000) Dietary genistein inactivates rat thyroid peroxidase in vivo without an apparent hypothyroid effect. *Toxicol. Appl. Pharmacol.*, **168**, 244–52.

Dalais, F.S., Rice, G.E., Wahlqvist, M.L. *et al.* (1998) Effects of dietary phytoestrogens in postmenopausal women. *Climacteric*, **1**, 124–9.

Divi, R.L. & Doerge, D.R. (1996) Inhibition of thyroid peroxidase by dietary flavonoids. *Chem. Res. Toxicol.*, **9**, 16–23.

Divi, R.L., Chang, H.C. & Doerge, D.R. (1997) Anti-thyroid isoflavones from soybean: isolation, characterisation, and mechanism of action. *Biochem. Pharmacol.*, **54**, 1087–96.

Duncan, A.M., Merz, B.E., Xu, X., Nagel, T.C., Phypps, W.R. & Kurzer, M.S. (1999a) Soy isoflavones exert modest effects in premenopausal women. *J. Clin. Endocrinol. Metab.*, **84**, 192–7.

Duncan, A.M., Underhill, K.E.W., Xu, X., Lavalleur, J., Phipps, W.R. & Kurzer, M.S. (1999b) Modest hormonal effects of soy isoflavones in postmenopausal women. *J. Clin. Endocrinol. Metab.*, **84**, 3479–84.

Graves, A.B., Larson, E.B., Edland, S.D. *et al.* (1996) Prevalence of dementia and its subtypes in the Japanese American population of King country, Washinghton state. *Am. J. Epidemiol.*, **144**, 760–61.

Ichinowatari, N., Tatsunuma, T. & Makyiya, H. (1987) Epidemiological study of old age mental disorders in the two rural area of Japan. *Japan Journal of Psychiatry and Neurology*, **41**, 629-36.

Knight, D.C., Howes, J.B. & Eden, J.A. (1999) The effects of Promensil™ an isoflavone extract on menopausal symptoms. *Climacteric*, **2**, 79-84.

Kotsopoulus, D., Dalais, F.S., Liang, Y.L., McGrath, P.B. & Teede, H.J. (2000) The effects of soy protein containing phytoestrogens on menopausal symptoms on postmenopausal women. *Climacteric*, **316**, 161-7.

Kuiper, G., Lemmen, J., Carlsson, B.O. *et al.* (1998) Interaction of estrogen chemical and phytoestrogen with estrogen receptor β. *Endocrinology*, **39**, 4552-63.

Murkies, A.L., Lombard, C., Strauss, B.J.G., Wilkox, G., Burger, H.G. & Morton, M.S. (1995) Dietary flower supplementation decreases post-menopausal hot flushes: effect of soy and wheat. *Maturitas*, **21**, 189-95.

Pan, Y., Antony, M., Watson, S. & Clarckson, T.B. (2000) Soy phytoestrogens improve radial arm maze performance in ovariectomized retired breeder rats and do not attenuate benefit of 17β-estrdiol treatment. *Menopause*, **7**, 230-35.

Parkin, D.M., Pisani, P. & Ferlay, J. (1993) Estimates of the world wide incidence of eighteen major cancers in 1985. *Int. J. Cancer*, **54**, 594-606.

Potter, S.N., Baum, J.A., Teng, H., Stillman, R.J., Shay, N.F. & Erdman, J.W. (1998) Soy protein and isoflavones: their effects on blood lipids and bone density in postmenopausal women. *Am. J. Clin. Nutr.*, **68**, 1375S-79S.

Quella, S.K., Loprinzi, C.L., Barton, D.L. *et al.* (2000) Evaluation of soy phytoestrogens for the treatment of hot flushes in breast cancer survivors: a north central cancer treatment group trial. *J. Clin. Oncol.*, **18**, 1068-74.

Scambia, G., Mango, D., Signorile, P.G. *et al.* (2000) Clinical effects of a standardized soy extract in postmenopasual women: a pilot study. *Menopause*, **2**, 105-11.

Upmalis, D.H., Lobo, R., Bradley, L., Warren, M., Cone, F.C. & Lamia, C.A. (2000) Vasomotor symptoms relief by soy isoflavone extract tablets in post-menopausal women; a multicenter, double-blind, randomized, placebo-controlled study. *Menopause*, **7**, 236-42.

Washburn, S., Burke, G.L., Morgan, T. & Antony, M. (1999) Effect of soy protein supplementation on serum lipoproteins, blood pressure, and menopausal symptoms in perimenopausal women. *Menopause*, **6**, 7-13.

Wilcox, G., Wahquist, M.L., Burger, H. & Medley, G. (1990) Oestrogenic effects of plant food in postmenopausal women. *BMJ*, **301**, 905-6.

INDEX

**Mars Confectionery was proud to support the first
Nutrition and Health Conference**

Visitors to our stand in the exhibition were able to find
out more about nutrition for sport and to learn about
the benefits of chocolate in a healthy balanced diet.

If you missed your chance, why not visit
the Chocolate Information Centre at :
www.chocolateinfo.com

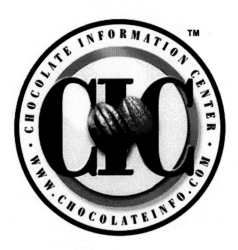

Or write to us at :
External Affairs, Mars Confectionery, SLOUGH, SL1 4JX
for details of our sports nutrition library

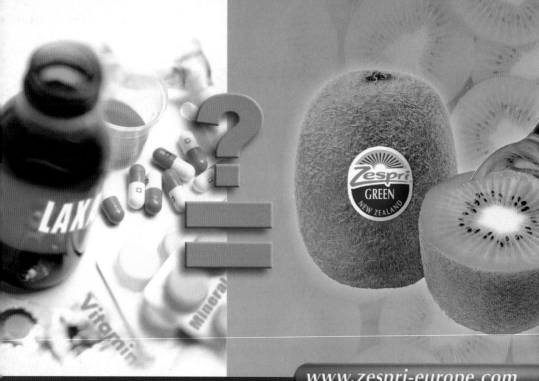

Nature at its best

Kiwifruit	16		
Papaya - Lemon Strawberry	14	13	12
Mango - Orange Banana	12	11	4
Grape - Pear Nectarine Apple	4	3	2	2

Nutrient density index = the daily value (dv) per 100g : an index that expresses the capacity of the fruit to serve the daily recommended quantities for the 9 most important nutrients.

Eating vegetables and fruit regularly contributes to a healthy, balanced diet.

The importance of kiwis in the daily fruit basket has been made clear by a scientific study carried out by Dr. Paul LaChance of the Department of Food Science and Nutrition of the Rutgers University in New Jersey (USA), in which 27 readily available varieties of fruit were compared.

He came to the conclusion that the kiwi – per 100g - supplies more nutrients to the body than any other kind of popular fruit.

One kiwi per day consequently makes many expensive, synthetic vitamin preparations and food supplements superfluous.

ZESPRI Service Centre, De Keyserlei 5, B-2018 Antwerpen

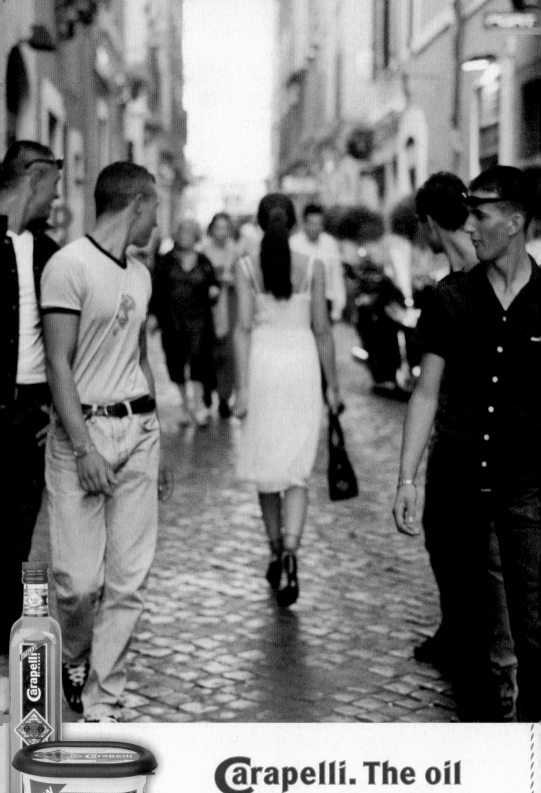

Carapelli. The oil that fuels Italians.

MARKS & SPENCER'S NUTRITIONAL MISSION

Marks & Spencer is dedicated to researching, developing and providing the highest quality healthy food ranges and helping people to make informed choices on good health and nutrition.

The retailer has a special Health & Wellbeing team that works with nutritionists and health care experts to develop innovative, healthy and great tasting food ranges.

As a one-brand retailer, Marks & Spencer can also set the standard for all its food products to make sure they adhere to strict policies on ingredient integrity and are nutritionally balanced to meet its exclusive standards. For example, did you know that the salt levels have been reduced in foods to ensure the salt content takes heed of UK Government recommendations?

The Health & Wellbeing team also ensures that customers get clear and concise information through accurate on-pack labelling. Nutritional information panels show sodium as salt equivalent, while a Guideline Daily Amount panel indicates the Recommended Daily Amount of calories, fat and salt for males and females and how much a portion contributes to a persons' total daily diet. A 'contains box' is also featured listing common allergens and support literature is offered to health care professionals to clearly explain the nutritional messages.

The team works with a number of organisations on awareness raising projects. In June this year, Marks & Spencer joined forces with the British Dietetic Association for the launch of 'Give Me Five' – a nationwide campaign that was promoted throughout Marks & Spencer's 297 stores to encourage more people to eat the recommended daily five portions of fruit and vegetables.